Adherence in Dermatology

Scott A. Davis

Editor

Adherence in Dermatology

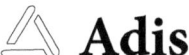

Editor
Scott A. Davis
Eshelman School of Pharmacy, CB#7355
University of North Carolina
Chapel Hill, NC
USA

ISBN 978-3-319-30992-7   ISBN 978-3-319-30994-1   (eBook)
DOI 10.1007/978-3-319-30994-1

Library of Congress Control Number: 2016940097

Printed on acid-free paper

This Adis imprint is published by Springer Nature
The registered company is Springer International Publishing AG Switzerland

Acknowledgments

I would like to thank the team at Springer for all the help and encouragement in writing this book, particularly Dene Peters for inviting me to write it. I would like to thank Prasad Gurunadham and Cameron Wright for all their wonderful assistance.

I would like to thank the Royster Society of Fellows at UNC Chapel Hill for giving me the protected time to work on this project during the summer of 2015.

I would like to acknowledge my professors, including Jenny Lund, Stacie Dusetzina, Til Stürmer, Gang Fang, Joel Farley, Daniel Westreich, Carol Golin, and Sue Blalock. I would also like to thank Betsy Sleath and Delesha Carpenter for their great mentorship since I have joined their team.

I would like to thank all my colleagues for their great insights and encouragement over the years, especially Karen Huang, Irma Richardson, Alan Fleischer, Amy McMichael, and Robert Anderson. Extra-special thanks to Steve Feldman for reviewing all my chapters and for giving me all the opportunities to grow as a researcher over the past few years. I would also like to thank Galderma Laboratories, L.P., for continued support of our research since 2003.

I would like to thank my family, Jim and Jean Davis.

Contents

Part I
What Is Known About
Adherence Behavior

Chapter 1
Impact of Nonadherence in Dermatology

Nazmine Sohi and Scott A. Davis

Nonadherence is ubiquitous in the field of dermatology. The importance of it is demonstrated with how impactful it is in the practice setting. For example, the effectiveness of scientifically proven treatment protocols and the presence of certain side effects are contingent upon adherence [1, 2]. However, there is a disconnect between physicians and proper knowledge over adherence. Along with having limited time to address and prioritize the issue, physicians may not have the correct training or background on the subject [3]. Medical education generally falls short with preparing physicians in different social and behavioral matters. There are proven risk factors to be aware of within the patient population which contribute to lower adherence: a patient's level of concern for treatment, the quality of a patient-physician relationship, and existing patient depression/psychosocial problems [3].

1.1 Clinical Impact

In order to provide the best clinical care possible, healthcare providers need to be aware of patient adherence. Tracking adherence allows us to accurately assume whether or not a treatment was effective. Physicians should understand the difference between treatment outcomes in clinical trials in comparison to the outcomes in practice [4]. Clinical trials show better results for medications due to higher adherence [4]. Failure to acknowledge this relationship may cause clinicians to assume

N. Sohi
Department of Dermatology, Wake Forest School of Medicine, Winston-Salem, NC, USA

S.A. Davis (✉)
Department of Dermatology, Wake Forest School of Medicine, Winston-Salem, NC, USA

Division of Pharmaceutical Outcomes and Policy, University of North Carolina Eshelman School of Pharmacy, Chapel Hill, NC, USA
e-mail: sdavis81@email.unc.edu

© Springer International Publishing Switzerland 2016
S.A. Davis (ed.), *Adherence in Dermatology*,
DOI 10.1007/978-3-319-30994-1_1

that tachyphylaxis has occurred – that the patient developed tolerance to the medication and thus it did not work as well. Actually, the patient may simply be showing lower adherence over time, so the assumption of tachyphylaxis would falsely influence practice decisions [5]. Physicians may erroneously characterize the patient as sensitive, the treatment as ineffective, or the treatment as primary cause of side effects [5].

More seriously, not adhering to physician's instructions unnecessarily puts patients at greater risks. For example, it was reported that only about 30 % of adults properly engage in skin-protective practices [6]. This type of nonadherence increases a patient's risk for skin cancer [6]. For diseases like psoriasis that require long-term care, nonadherence has a significant effect on the severity of symptoms present, different treatment outcomes, and the quality of life [7, 8]. Related to the high rates of nonadherence, an estimated 52.3 % of patients with psoriasis report being disappointed with their treatment [9]. This disappointment is not inevitable; as we shall see in this book, there is much that can be done. However, first it is necessary to realize that the patient is disappointed in some way with the regimen and would welcome changes that would make the treatment more satisfactory.

1.2   Economic Impact

When considering the healthcare system at large, nonadherence is linked to higher associated costs [3]. Overall, as much as $100 billion is spent on hospitalizations that could have been prevented with better medication adherence [10]. In a study done on Crohn's disease patients, nonadherence was correlated with higher incidences of hospitalizations, increasing adjusted hospitalization costs as high as 115 % ($9,570–$11,450) [11]. Additionally, this study demonstrated how nonadherence caused a 90 % ($4,961) increase in medical-related costs for Crohn's disease [11]. Another study assessing the return on investment of better medication adherence in diabetes, hypertension, and hyperlipidemia found that each dollar spent on medications resulted in a savings on medical costs of $4 in hypertension, $5 in hyperlipidemia, and $7 in diabetes [12, 13]. Although similar data are not yet available in dermatology, it would not be surprising that the costs of dermatological treatments and drugs might also be higher with higher nonadherence rates. Future research needs to address this gap in the literature.

1.3   Magnitude

Lack of adherence is relevant to discuss in dermatology because it is evidently widespread [9]. In the field of dermatology, a reported range of 30–80 % of patients admit to nonadherence at some point in their care plan [7]. For example, about 40 % of psoriasis patients and 23.7 % of acne patients are nonadherent [14, 15]. When considering different sexes or age groups, lack of adherence is found to be a common, nondiscriminatory problem that affects all types of patients [1]. There is a certain amount of variation, with adolescents typically being the least adherent, but all patients are susceptible to adherence issues (see Chap. 3).

Healthcare professionals are in a position to confront and correct the gaps in care that nonadherence creates. Knowledge on how to educate and support patients correctly has the potential to change these disappointing statistics [9]. There is not yet a guide available that addresses adherence in dermatology. This book will provide you with the right tools and resources to become aware of an overlooked, yet critical issue in practice.

References

1. Anderson KL, Dothard EH, Huang KE, Feldman SR (2015) Frequency of primary nonadherence to acne treatment. JAMA Dermatol 151(6):623–626
2. Peris K, Neri L, Fargnoli MC, Pellacani G (2014) Physicians' concerns towards prescription adherence and treatment effectiveness in the clinical management of actinic keratosis. G Ital Dermatol Venereol 149(2):193–198
3. Vangeli E, Bakhshi S, Baker A et al (2015) A systematic review of factors associated with non-adherence to treatment for immune-mediated inflammatory diseases. Adv Ther 32(11):983–1028
4. Davis SA, Feldman SR (2013) Using Hawthorne effects to improve adherence in clinical practice: lessons from clinical trials. JAMA Dermatol 149(4):490–491
5. Nolan BV, Feldman SR (2009) Adherence, the fourth dimension in the geometry of dermatological treatment. Arch Dermatol 145(11):1319–1321
6. Buller DB, Cokkinides V, Hall HI et al (2011) Prevalence of sunburn, sun protection, and indoor tanning behaviors among Americans: review from national surveys and case studies of 3 states. J Am Acad Dermatol 65(5 Suppl 1):S114–S123
7. Evers AW, Kleinpenning MM, Smits T et al (2010) Treatment nonadherence and long-term effects of narrowband UV-B therapy in patients with psoriasis. Arch Dermatol 146(2):198–199
8. Thorneloe RJ, Bundy C, Griffiths CE, Ashcroft DM, Cordingley L (2013) Adherence to medication in patients with psoriasis: a systematic literature review. Br J Dermatol 168(1):20–31
9. Armstrong AW, Robertson AD, Wu J, Schupp C, Lebwohl MG (2013) Undertreatment, treatment trends, and treatment dissatisfaction among patients with psoriasis and psoriatic arthritis in the United States: findings from the National Psoriasis Foundation surveys, 2003–2011. JAMA Dermatol 149(10):1180–1185
10. Osterberg L, Blaschke T (2005) Adherence to medication. N Engl J Med 353:487–497
11. Kane SV, Chao J, Mulani PM (2009) Adherence to infliximab maintenance therapy and health care utilization and costs by Crohn's disease patients. Adv Ther 26(10):936–946
12. Logan T The future of community pharmacy: star ratings, medication adherence, and community pharmacy's evolving role. Available at http://www.asapnet.org/files/January2014/Presentations/ASAPJan14_Presentations08_Logan1.pdf. Accessed 26 Dec 2015
13. Sokol MC, McGuigan KA, Verbrugge RR, Epstein RS (2005) Impact of medication adherence on hospitalization risk and healthcare cost. Med Care 43:521–530
14. Richards HL, Fortune DG, Griffiths CE (2006) Adherence to treatment in patients with psoriasis. J Eur Acad Dermatol Venereol 20(4):370–379
15. Snyder S, Crandell I, Davis SA, Feldman SR (2014) Medical adherence to acne therapy: a systematic review. Am J Clin Dermatol 15(2):87–94

Chapter 2
Models of Adherence

Imran Aslam, Michael E. Farhangian, and Steven R. Feldman

Whether patients take their medication is determined by a myriad of factors ranging from socioeconomic factors to disease-related issues [20]. While many of these factors are immutable by the dermatologist, having a solid understanding of what internally drives patients to engage in health-seeking behavior can be instrumental in tackling adherence problems. Adherence models are theoretical constructs that have been created to help further elucidate the complexities of what drives patients to adhere to their medications. These models provide a framework for which interventions can be developed to target the major determining factors that can adversely affect adherence to medication.

There are many models of adherence that have been developed. These models of adherence have been categorized into (1) biomedical, (2) behavioral, (3) communication, (4) cognitive, and (5) self-regulatory in addition to the more recent transtheoretical model (Table 2.1) [16, 20]. The transtheoretical and cognitive models are most commonly used to rationalize adherence behavior [20].

2.1 Types of Adherence Models

2.1.1 Biomedical Models

The biomedical models are some of the more primitive models of adherence. They characterize the patients as beings with an illness who are passively accepting treatment from their provider. They rationalize a patient's difficulties with adhering to their medication as being due to their intrinsic personality deficits. This type of adherence model ignores the dynamic nature of the individual and isolates

I. Aslam • M.E. Farhangian • S.R. Feldman (✉)
Department of Dermatology, Wake Forest School of Medicine, Winston-Salem, NC, USA
e-mail: sfeldman@wakehealth.edu

© Springer International Publishing Switzerland 2016
S.A. Davis (ed.), *Adherence in Dermatology*,
DOI 10.1007/978-3-319-30994-1_2

Table 2.1 Models of adherence

Models of adherence	Overview	Pros	Cons
Biomedical	Emphasizes that patients are passive recipients of treatment	Leads to advances in adherence research [16]	Ignores basic social and psychological factors that influence adherence [16]
Behavioral	Past experiences dictate adherence behaviors	Using rewards can help implement positive lifestyle changes and improve adherence to medication [16]	Ignores the less conscious reasons that influence patient adherence that are not linked to immediate rewards [3] Not effective in producing long-term behavior change [16]
Communication	Emphasizes the importance of communicating clear, specific instructions	Effective communication can be a simple means of improving adherence	Certain instances exist where proper communication does not improve adherence [16]
Self-regulatory	Emotional influences and cognitive reasoning are parallel processes that determine patient's behavior	Accounts for both emotional and cognitive influences in explaining patient's behavior	Little supporting data and difficult to use in studies because of multivariate nature [16]
Transtheoretical	Presents behavior change as a series of stages	Important to tailor approach to behavior change by first identifying an individual's stage	Ignores social context of change, i.e., socioeconomic status Differentiation between the stages can be arbitrary, because there are no set criteria to determine an individual's stage of change
Cognitive	Adherence is directly related to an individual's attitudes, beliefs, and expectations regarding treatment	Focuses on the conscious, intentional decision-making [16]	Does not adequately address the automatic, habitual behaviors such as smoking and eating [16]

adherence problems from the social contexts that often play a large role [3]. This model attempts to overcome poor adherence by identifying individuals who have personality traits that puts them at risk for poor adherence [3]. Although there are certain personalities that predispose to poor adherence, the biomedical model doesn't take into account the many other drivers of poor adherence that are not personality "faults," such as financial burden and social factors such as the relationship between the provider and the patient [16, 20, 28].

2.1.2 Behavioral Models

Behavioral models of adherence speak more to learned behavior being the cause of poor adherence [16]. This is in contrast to the biomedical model; rather than an individual's personality traits leading to poor adherence, it instead focuses on one's life experiences as the predominant influence on adherence behavior. Fundamentally, this model of adherence is rooted in the understanding that patient's adherence patterns are learned through their past experiences (which can be thoughts or external cues) and their subsequent association with either positive or negative stimuli [20]. Through this understanding, rewarding patients has been used to help patients associate their adherence to medication with a positive stimulus [16].

2.1.3 Communication Models

The communication models emphasize the importance of discussing general information about illness and treatment options and communicating clear, specific instructions that are at the level of the patient's understanding [16]. Many instances of poor patient adherence can be attributed to poor communication between the provider and patient. It is the responsibility of the caregiver to ensure that the patient understands his condition and the respective treatment. Once the instructions are communicated properly, then it is up to the patient to decide if he would like to accept it or not. This acceptance process is strongly influenced by the caregiver's persuasion capabilities as well as the underlying provider-patient relationship [16].

2.1.4 Transtheoretical Model

The transtheoretical model explains behavior change as a progression of five stages: precontemplation, contemplation, preparation, action, and maintenance. The first stage, precontemplation, is the period in which an individual is not considering any change in the next 6 months. Contemplation is when the individual initially starts to consider changing a behavior sometime in the next 6 months. The third stage is preparation which is when an individual is preparing for a change in the next month. During the preparation stage, individuals typically have a plan of action such as joining a gym or getting a fitness coach. The fourth stage is action. During this phase an individual is actively engaging in behavior change. Maintenance is the last stage that typically begins 6 months after the action stage. The goal of this stage is to maintain the behavior change and avoid relapse. Overall the transtheoretical model presents behavior change as a process and emphasizes the individual's intentions and decision-making [1, 14].

2.1.5 Cognitive

The cognitive model indicates that adherence is directly related to an individual's attitudes, beliefs, and expectations regarding treatment [26]. The assumption is that if patients understand and are able to weigh the advantages and risks of treatment, they will be more likely to adhere [26]. Examples of cognitive theories include the health belief model, protection motivation theory, social cognitive theory, and theory of planned behavior. The health belief model will be discussed in further detail in the following section.

2.1.6 Self-Regulatory

The self-regulatory model also accounts for cognitive factors, but in addition it also considers emotional factors as well. The patient's perception of his illness is determined by external stimuli (physician advice, media health messages) and internal stimuli (patient's own symptoms). These stimuli elicit both cognitive and emotional reactions that collectively influence the patient's behavior. An example of how emotions can influence healthcare decisions is when a woman's fear of having breast cancer inhibits her from getting a mammogram [16]. Furthermore, this model explains why people can view the same illness differently in a cognitive fashion as well as react differently emotionally [16].

2.2 Behavioral Economics and Adherence

Most of these traditional adherence models that we have discussed are very rationalistic and deterministic. With the exception of the self-regulatory model, these traditional rational choice models do not account for instances in which there is a deviation from rational thinking. Advances in behavioral economics have demonstrated that this deviation from rational thought processes occurs much more commonly than we once thought. For instance, a patient's perception of their medication will differ depending on whether the physician says, "Taking this will make you live a year longer" versus "Not taking this will make you die a year earlier." This is a simple example of a principle called loss aversion which describes how humans are more likely to take action in order to avoid a loss rather than to acquire a gain [12]. Cognitive biases such as loss aversion describe tendencies in human thinking that lead to irrational decisions and behaviors. There are a number of cognitive biases studied in behavioral economics, and it is important to consider the influence of these principles when discussing patient adherence [12].

2.3   Why Is a Model Important

While the principles of behavioral economics have challenged our thinking about adherence, the traditional models are still important. A conceptual model to understand adherence is very valuable because it helps us understand the mechanism of how an intervention targets the root cause of poor adherence, rather than just blindly trying out an intervention and seeing what happens. Conceptual models are a great tool to use when developing, assessing, and evaluating interventions aimed at improving adherence. This is especially true considering that many interventions attempting to improve adherence fail [15]. The health belief model (HBM) is the most commonly used model and has demonstrated success in predicting health behavior [10].

2.4   The Health Belief Model

The underlying principle of the HBM is that patients weigh the benefits versus the barriers to treatment when deciding whether or not to adhere. The HBM conceptualizes patient adherence based on six components. The decision to partake in a health-related behavior is based on an individual's (1) perceived susceptibility, (2) perceived severity, (3) perceived benefit, (4) perceived barriers, (5) cues to action, and (6) self-efficacy (Table 2.2) [10]. In a review of HBM studies, perceived barriers and perceived benefits had the greatest influence on health behaviors, while perceived severity had the weakest influence [4, 10].

Table 2.2 Adherence interventions

HBM components	Interventions
Perceived susceptibility/severity	Pt education on nature of disease:
	Informational workbooks [24]
	Handouts
	Educational websites
	Informational YouTube videos
Perceived benefit	Pt education on effectiveness of therapy [18]
	Provide goals for therapy
Perceived barriers	Determine potential barriers to therapy
	Provide affordable treatments [13]
Cues to action	Audiovisual reminder system [5]
	Telephone calls
	Reminder packaging
Self-efficacy	Motivational interviewing [7]

2.4.1 Perceived Susceptibility

Perceived susceptibility refers to the extent to which a person feels that they are at risk for contracting an illness or disease. The more susceptible a patient feels to a certain illness, the more likely that person is to accept and seek treatment for that illness. If a patient has a relative with skin cancer, he may feel more susceptible to developing skin cancer and consequently be more likely to consider getting a skin exam. Educational interventions are useful in making patients aware of their risk of developing certain conditions. For example, kidney transplant patients are at a higher risk of developing skin cancer due to antirejection medications. Consequently researchers designed an informational workbook that educated patients on how antirejection medications increase the risk of developing squamous cell carcinoma (SCC) of the skin, the importance of early detection, and how to recognize the early warning signs of SCCs [24]. Participants who received this workbook demonstrated a better understanding of their risk and were more likely to perform self skin exams and see a dermatologist if they noticed anything concerning [24].

2.4.2 Perceived Severity

Perceived severity is a patient's understanding of just how serious their disease is. If a patient does not believe that their illness is severe, they may not feel that it warrants treatment and may not be adherent to the treatment that they are being provided. In addition to perceived susceptibility, a patient will be further motivated to seek and adhere to treatment if he/she understands and is concerned about the potential severity of the disease. For instance, a patient may be more likely to use sunscreen daily if they understand that they might lose their life from skin cancer if they fail to protect their skin from the sun. Many adherence interventions incorporate education on the complications that can arise from poor management of disease, in an attempt to convey to patients the severity of their illness. Adherence interventions aimed at improving asthma management include educating patients on the effects of asthma can have on sleep, physical activity, potential for hospitalizations, and even death [27]. Similarly for diabetes, researchers educated patients on the many complications that can arise from uncontrolled glucose levels [19].

Perceived severity may have unexpected effects. Greater perceived severity does not necessarily imply that patients will be more likely to use their medication. Patients may be so bothered by the disease as not to want to even think about it. In such cases, medication may not be taken because it would serve to remind the patient about their psychically painful condition.

2.4.3   Perceived Benefits

The benefits of treatment should be made clear to patients in order to improve adherence. For instance, if a patient is not convinced that the skin exam is a good screening tool for skin cancer, they are unlikely to see their dermatologist for skin exams. Interventions that help patients weigh the risks and benefits of a medication significantly improve patient adherence [18, 22]. As part of an intervention to improve adherence to highly active antiretroviral therapy (HAART), patients that were educated on the risk and benefits of treatment had higher adherence rates than patients that received standard care [22]. Another way to encourage patients is to provide them with goals of therapy. For instance, providers may tell patients they can expect a 75 % improvement in their rash over the next 2 weeks of treatment. While it can be difficult for providers to anticipate how a patient will respond to therapy, an estimation that under promises and over delivers may help motivate patients.

2.4.4   Perceived Barriers

Perceived barriers encompass all of the things that an individual views as a hurdle to behavior change. There are many barriers that make it difficult for patients to engage in health-promoting behavior. Some examples of barriers to getting a skin exam include time, money, and embarrassment. Getting a skin exam can be costly in terms of time and money especially if the patient has to take time off work. Furthermore, patients may feel embarrassed by their physical appearance and may not feel comfortable getting a skin exam. Interventions to overcome these barriers can help improve adherence. A home-based nursing intervention that included working with patients directly to identify and address perceived barriers was successful in improving adherence to antiretroviral therapy [2]. Cost of treatment is another potential barrier for medications with high co-payments that were associated with poor adherence [13]. Therefore providers should be aware of cheaper alternative therapies or provide patients with information on potential coverage programs.

2.4.5   Cues to Action

Cues to action are reminders for patients to perform a health behavior. These cues can be internal or external. Internal cues could be patient's symptoms like a tender skin lesion that reminds an individual to get a skin exam or they can be external which may take the form of health messages, such as an article encouraging readers to have screening tests done. When medications are irritating, the irritation may act as a cue to use treatment; more tolerable treatments do not automatically result in better adherence than less tolerable treatments [8].

External reminders can come in many forms but a few examples include telephone calls, text messages, and reminder packaging. In an effort to improve adherence to inhaled corticosteroid (ICS) therapy, researchers integrated an audiovisual reminder system into the inhaler that acts as an alarm system and beeps whenever a dose is due and also provides a visual cue to show the user if they have taken their inhaler during a certain period of time [5]. This innovative device successfully improved patient adherence to ICS therapy and has the potential to be incorporated into other therapies as well [5]. Other reminder strategies such as text messages have demonstrated mixed results with some studies reporting that they helped to improve adherence while others reporting that they did not [9, 25, 29].

2.4.6 Self-Efficacy

Self-efficacy is an element of the HBM that was added in years after its inception [6, 23]. It refers to the patients' faith in their abilities to overcome their condition. An example of self-efficacy is "Do I have the discipline to put on sunscreen before I go outside every day?" Interventions such as motivational interviewing (MI) is a means of improving self-efficacy and has demonstrated some success in promoting positive health behaviors [7, 11]. MI is a unique style of patient-centered counseling that utilizes a series of directed questions to help patients reach a specific conclusion and plan of action [17]. MI allows patients to come up with their "own" solutions and in doing so improve self-efficacy. MI techniques have been used to improve adherence rates among patients on HAART [7].

2.5 Conclusion

Patient adherence is a very relevant and important topic in healthcare. It is estimated that about 20–50 % of patients do not take their medication as prescribed [15]. As we have discussed earlier, there are numerous models that contribute to our understanding of patient adherence. These models are essential when developing, assessing, and evaluating interventions aimed at improving adherence. They provide a conceptual framework that helps researchers employ effective interventions and also enables practitioners to understand the nuances of adherence. While no model is perfect, the HBM is among the most widely used [10]. Patient adherence is a multifaceted issue, and interventions designed to improve adherence hold the most potential when they address all or multiple components of the HBM.

References

1. Armitage CJ, Conner M (2000) Social cognition models and health behaviour: a structured review. Psychol Health 15(2):173–189
2. Berrien VM, Salazar JC, Reynolds E, McKay K (2004) Adherence to antiretroviral therapy in HIV-infected pediatric patients improves with home-based intensive nursing intervention. AIDS Patient Care STDS 18(6):355–363
3. Blackwell B (1992) Compliance. Psychother Psychosom 58(3–4):161–169
4. Carpenter CJ (2010) A meta-analysis of the effectiveness of health belief model variables in predicting behavior. Health Commun 25(8):661–669
5. Charles T, Quinn D, Weatherall M, Aldington S, Beasley R, Holt S (2007) An audiovisual reminder function improves adherence with inhaled corticosteroid therapy in asthma. J Allergy Clin Immunol 119(4):811–816
6. Clark NM, Rosenstock IM, Hassan H, Evans D, Wasilewski Y, Feldman C, Mellins RB (1988) The effect of health beliefs and feelings of self efficacy on self management behavior of children with a chronic disease. Patient Educ Couns 11(2):131–139. doi:10.1016/0738-3991 (88)90045-6
7. DiIorio C, Resnicow K, McDonnell M, Soet J, McCarty F, Yeager K (2003) Using motivational interviewing to promote adherence to antiretroviral medications: a pilot study. J Assoc Nurses AIDS Care 14(2):52–62
8. Feldman SR (2008) Practical ways to improve patients' treatment outcomes. Medical Quality Enhancement Corporation, Winston-Salem, North Carolina
9. Foreman KF, Stockl KM, Le LB, Fisk E, Shah SM, Lew HC, Solow BK, Curtis BS (2012) Impact of a text messaging pilot program on patient medication adherence. Clin Ther 34(5):1084–1091
10. Glanz K, Rimer BK, Viswanath K (2008) Health behavior and health education: theory, research, and practice. Wiley, San Francisco
11. Holstad MM, DiIorio C, Kelley ME, Resnicow K, Sharma S (2011) Group motivational interviewing to promote adherence to antiretroviral medications and risk reduction behaviors in HIV infected women. AIDS Behav 15(5):885–896
12. Kahneman D (2011) Thinking, fast and slow. Farrar, Straus, & Giroux, New York.
13. Kessler RC, Cantrell CR, Berglund P, Sokol MC (2007) The effects of copayments on medication adherence during the first two years of prescription drug treatment. J Occup Environ Med 49(6):597–609
14. Kowalski K, Jeznach A, Tuokko HA (2014) Stages of driving behavior change within the Transtheoretical Model (TM). J Safety Res 50:17–25
15. Kripalani S, Yao X, Haynes RB (2007) Interventions to enhance medication adherence in chronic medical conditions: a systematic review. Arch Intern Med 167(6):540–550
16. Leventhal H, Cameron L (1987) Behavioral theories and the problem of compliance. Patient Educ Couns 10(2):117–138. doi:10.1016/0738-3991(87)90093-0
17. Markland D, Ryan RM, Tobin VJ, Rollnick S (2005) Motivational interviewing and self–determination theory. J Soc Clin Psychol 24(6):811–831
18. Marquez Contreras E, Vegazo Garcia O, Martel Claros N, Gil Guillen V, de la Figuera von Wichmann M, Casado Martinez JJ, Fernandez R (2005) Efficacy of telephone and mail intervention in patient compliance with antihypertensive drugs in hypertension. ETECUM-HTA study. Blood Press 14(3):151–158
19. Mazroui A, Rashid N, Kamal MM, Ghabash NM, Yacout TA, Kole PL, McElnay JC (2009) Influence of pharmaceutical care on health outcomes in patients with type 2 diabetes mellitus. Br J Clin Pharmacol 67(5):547–557
20. Munro SA, Lewin SA, Smith HJ, Engel ME, Fretheim A, Volmink J (2007) Patient adherence to tuberculosis treatment: a systematic review of qualitative research. PLoS Med 4(7):e238
21. World Health Organization, Sabaté E (2003) Adherence to long-term therapies: evidence for action. World Health Organization, Geneva

22. Pearson CR, Micek MA, Simoni JM, Hoff PD, Matediana E, Martin DP, Gloyd SS (2007) Randomized control trial of peer-delivered, modified directly observed therapy for HAART in Mozambique. J Acquir Immune Defic Syndr 46(2):238–244
23. Riekert KA, Ockene JK, Pbert L, Ebooks Corporation (2013) The handbook of health behavior change, Springer, NYC, NY
24. Robinson JK, Turrisi R, Mallett KA, Stapleton J, Boone SL, Kim N, Riyat NV, Gordon EJ (2011) Efficacy of an educational intervention with kidney transplant recipients to promote skin self-examination for squamous cell carcinoma detection. Arch Dermatol 147(6):689–695
25. Tran N, Coffman JM, Sumino K, Cabana MD (2014) Patient reminder systems and asthma medication adherence: a systematic review. J Asthma 51(5):536–43
26. Unni EJ (2008) Development of models to predict medication non-adherence based on a new typology. ProQuest, Iowa
27. Wang K-Y, Chian C-F, Lai H-R, Tarn Y-H, Wu C-P (2010) Clinical pharmacist counseling improves outcomes for Taiwanese asthma patients. Pharm World Sci 32(6):721–729
28. Wu JR, Moser DK (2014) Type D personality predicts poor medication adherence in patients with heart failure in the USA. Int J Behav Med 21(5):833–842
29. Yentzer BA, Gosnell AL, Clark AR, Pearce DJ, Balkrishnan R, Camacho FT, Young TA, Fountain JM, Fleischer AB Jr, Colón LE (2011) A randomized controlled pilot study of strategies to increase adherence in teenagers with acne vulgaris. J Am Acad Dermatol 64(4):793–795

Chapter 3
Impact of Demographic and Treatment-Related Factors

Ruth Blair and Girish Gupta

3.1 Introduction

Compliance is now considered an out-of-date term as it implies patients' inability or unwillingness to do what they are told by a learned professional. Compliance, or more so, the lack of compliance, is a negative term that should now be avoided. Concordance suggests the agreement of treatment type and regimen agreed by the health-care provider and the patient and is a positive ideal to be encouraged [1]. Adherence will be positively or negatively affected by the degree of concordance, thus highlighting the need for careful consideration by the health-care provider[1] of the individual needs of each patient and to encourage a holistic approach to patient management [2].

Adherence to treatment is important in all conditions but particularly so in chronic disease. A study by the World Health Organization estimated that only 50 % of patients with chronic disease in developed countries follow their treatment as recommended [1]. Patients with chronic diseases will require frequent, if not life-long, treatment and often in many forms. If adherence is good but that particular

---

[1] For the purposes of this chapter, the health-care provider denotes anyone involved in the care of patients with skin disease from the general practitioner and the dermatologist to the district and specialist nurses to the nursing assistants and students, to those involved in support groups and provision of patient information leaflets. Thus, when the term health-care provider, doctor or dermatologist is used, it should be taken to encompass all of the different members of this multidisciplinary team.

R. Blair
Department of Dermatology, Queen Elizabeth University Hospital,
Glasgow, Scotland

G. Gupta (✉)
Department of Dermatology, NHS Lanarkshire, Airdrie, Lanarkshire, Scotland
e-mail: Girish.Gupta@lanarkshire.scot.nhs.uk

© Springer International Publishing Switzerland 2016   17
S.A. Davis (ed.), *Adherence in Dermatology*,
DOI 10.1007/978-3-319-30994-1_3

treatment does not work, then the health-care provider can feel more confident in discontinuing the treatment and moving on to something else. However, if adherence is poor, then it can be difficult to assess the efficacy of treatment in that subject. This may result in an effective treatment being abandoned and permanently discontinued by both the patient and health-care provider in favour of something that may be more toxic or less efficacious.

The purpose of this chapter is to ascertain what factors affect adherence in dermatology patients via literature search. There is a wealth of information available on adherence issues in various skin conditions, and we have chosen to focus on the more common dermatoses.

3.2 Assessing Adherence

Assessing adherence in a clinical setting can be challenging. Patients may feel a sense of embarrassment admitting that they have not been using their treatment as prescribed. They may also feel that they have to apologise as if they have somehow let their health-care provider down. If patients do admit to poor adherence, then their honesty should be acknowledged, and the reason for not using the treatment should be sought and discussed in a non-confrontational manner. Failure to do this may lead to a breakdown in the relationship, thus reducing the chance of future good adherence.

In some circumstances, it can be relatively easy to check treatment adherence through therapeutic blood monitoring or urinary excretion of products of drug metabolism. Just because a patient receives their prescription on time, it does not necessarily mean that they are using the treatment. However, in the case of topical therapy, the health-care provider can get some idea of patient adherence by asking about quantities of creams or ointments being used over a certain period of time and how often repeat prescriptions are being requested.

3.2.1 Adherence Assessment Tools

There are some tools that can be used in dermatology to assess the impact of the disease and the severity. The Dermatology Life Quality Index (DLQI) can be used in most chronic skin diseases to assess the impact of the disease on the patient's quality of life. The DLQI score is subjective.

Assessing disease severity can be difficult to gauge exactly. In psoriasis, the Psoriasis Area and Severity Index (PASI) can be a useful tool. However, there is a certain degree of intra- and inter-observer variation.

Documenting the DLQI and PASI score at each clinic visit can be useful assessing patient response to treatment, but it does not always address adherence.

The following are different tools that have been used for adherence research [3] purposes (see Chaps. 5, 6 and 7), but their practicality in the normal everyday clinic is (in most examples) impractical:

Direct measures (e.g. blood test)
Patient self-reported measures (e.g. patient log or interview)
Pharmacy prescription refill records
Medication use through assessing weight of treatment or number in the case of oral treatment
Medication event monitoring system (MEMS) – electronic record of opening and closing of medication bottle cap

3.3 An Approach to Adherence Issues

When considering treatment adherence in dermatology, one has to address the different treatment modalities available: topical (including dressings), oral, subcutaneous, intravenous, phototherapy and surgical. What possible barriers to each treatment type may arise, and how much of this is down to the patient and how much to the health-care provider?

The responsibility for good adherence at the initiation of any treatment is in the hands of the health-care provider, but the agreement of the patient to this treatment type is essential. It is important to understand the patient as an individual and to know what aspects of their life may impact on their ability to adhere to certain treatment modalities. Examples of these are other diseases or disability, polypharmacy, occupation, living alone, lower socio-economic class, poverty [1], poor living conditions, literacy [4], family or caring commitments and hobbies. Also more negative lifestyle factors such as tobacco smoking, excessive alcohol intake and drug misuse and dependence. Gender does not appear to be relevant except in acne [5–11].

Adherence is affected in a variable manner by age: infants' adherence is dependent on their carers. With young children, their own feelings towards treatments and their willingness to allow its application is one part, and the other is that of the carers' ability to adhere to the regime; in teenagers, over both genders, there is a decrease in adherence rates which may be due to changing attitudes to their disease, and to their parents and with adults, it will depend on other factors such as their work schedule and caring commitments. The elderly may be more willing to use treatments but may be less able [12].

The patient's race/ethnicity is also important. A study in America revealed that Black Americans have the poorest adherence rate, followed by Latino, Hispanic and Mexican-Americans. White Americans and Japanese Americans had the highest adherence rates [13]. Another important factor to consider is their beliefs prior to treatment: Have they suffered adverse events in the past; have they read negative or misleading press about a therapy; are they scared about potential side effects?

All these issues need to be addressed prior to starting treatment. If the patient already envisages problems with adhering to treatment before they have embarked on the treatment, then this needs to be discussed carefully, and if there seems to be a real barrier to adherence with the treatment, then an alternative should be sought.

As dermatologists, we ask a lot of our patients in terms of adherence. We ask them to apply topical agents which may be time-consuming and messy. Sometimes they have to attend hospital frequently for blood tests or treatments such as ultraviolet B (UVB). With some treatments they need to abstain from alcohol, avoid the sun and avoid pregnancy. Sometimes the treatment regimes can be so complicated that we struggle to understand it ourselves, yet we bombard the patient with a list of commands about what goes where and when to step down or step up. Our support is vital from the outset, and giving clear verbal instructions, written instructions, demonstrations, a point-of-contact, support groups and follow-up shows the patient we are supporting them.

The timing and frequency of treatment are important for good adherence. Applying topical agents first thing in the morning could prove a challenge if there are others within the household to consider, for example, getting children ready for school. Does the treatment then need to dry before clothing can go on? Does the treatment influence what clothing can be worn? Is the treatment uncomfortable under clothing during the day, thus affecting work? In terms of frequency of application, it stands to reason that the more often we ask patients to apply their treatment, the less likely they are to fully adhere to the regime.

For those patients who need to attend hospital for treatment (e.g. phototherapy and leg ulcer dressings), time off work, help with children, or lifts to and from hospital may be required. Thus, the more often they need to attend, the more likely they are to have to cancel appointments. However, if they know that their treatment can be done in the shortest possible time, this is helpful because they then know what to tell their colleagues at work, friends and family members about the duration of each absence.

In the case of oral treatment, timing is particularly important if side effects are an issue: nausea associated with methotrexate and flushing and diarrhoea associated with fumaric acid esters. Thus, counselling patients about these side effects and, in the case of methotrexate, allowing them the day of the week that will be least disruptive (some patients like to be at home with little to do if they feel nauseous, whereas others may prefer to be at work and distracted from their symptoms) will aid in their adherence. Significant side effects from medication may stop a patient taking that drug altogether, so considering concomitant therapy, such as folic acid supplementation with methotrexate, may reduce these side effects and thus aid adherence [22].

A simple drug regime will be easier to adhere to than a complicated one, but one also has to consider other medications the patient may be on in terms of adding yet another drug to a complicated daily regime as well as drug interactions. Supplying drug treatment in the form of a "dosette" box will reduce the chance of incorrect medication being taken and increase adherence.

With biologic therapy, adherence is much better than with topical or oral therapy for psoriasis and particularly at initiation when the drugs are administered in a clinical setting. In the case of infliximab administered by the provider, adherence is almost 100 % and almost wholly reliant on the patient turning up for their appointment and the drug being available. With the tumour necrosis factor-α (TNF-α) inhibitors, the adherence rate is quoted as 66 % regardless of the specific drug (frequency of administration does not seem to be an important factor) [14]. Providing good education and addressing the patient's concerns about this class of drugs in terms of efficacy and safety and potential side effects are essential from the outset. Clear instruction on administration, particularly self-administration, should be provided by someone knowledgeable and experienced.

3.4   Adherence Issues in Dermatology: Specific Cases

There are vast array of dermatological diagnoses and thus treatment regimens. It would be impossible within this chapter to cover each and every diagnosis and its management problems and solutions. However, with such similarities in so much of dermatological treatment, a good working knowledge of the major pitfalls with adherence in the management of more common dermatoses is helpful in the approach to the majority of dermatological conditions.

Below, adherence issues within specific patient groups and dermatological conditions are considered.

3.4.1   Adherence Challenges in the Paediatric Population

Adherence rates to treatment in the paediatric population range from 11 % to 93 % (median rate 58 %) [15]. Within dermatology, there have been studies particularly looking at adherence in atopic dermatitis and acne. One article summarised the issues faced by the health-care provider in identifying reasons for poor adherence in children, age-specific challenges and ways to overcome these hurdles [16]. Drotar et al. [17] developed a conceptual model looking at the influences on adherence in paediatric treatment of asthma, but these factors can also be applied to chronic dermatological disease. They grouped together the following categories:

1. Family demographic characteristic and functioning:

   • Household income and level of parental education
   • The family routine and level of communication within the household
   • Race

2. Parental characteristics:

   • Psychological adjustment to their child's illness and their knowledge of the illness
   • Beliefs regarding health, illness and treatment

3. Child characteristics:

   - Age
   - Psychological adjustment to their illness and knowledge of the illness
   - Beliefs regarding health, illness and treatment

4. Health-care system and provider variables:

   - Quality of medical care
   - Access to medical care
   - Communication with child and family

5. Child health outcomes:

   - Symptom control
   - Health-care utilisation
   - Improvement or impairment on quality of life

The health-care provider must do their upmost to positively influence the factors which are within their control.

Looking specifically at the characteristics of the child, age is very important. In infancy, primary school age group and adolescence, there are multiple factors that will influence the ability and the desire to adhere to treatment. Interestingly, as children age, they tend to have an increased understanding of their disease and the reason for treatment, and yet they are less likely to adhere [18]. When the child is a baby, the responsibility lies with the carer. It is imperative that the carer is educated in treatment application and why the treatment is being used and to allay fears about possible side effects; otherwise, there may be reluctance on the part of the carer to adhere to the regime. In later infancy/early primary school years, the child may find having treatments applied uncomfortable or cumbersome. They may not wish to stand still and allow a carer to apply their treatments. As the child gets older, the responsibility for therapy gradually shifts from their parents to them. They may not adhere to treatment because it is difficult to apply. However, factors such as being like their peers and not wanting to "stand out" can negatively influence adherence. They may not want to use their treatments because their parent tells them to, thus asserting their own feelings of control [16].

So how can we improve treatment adherence in our paediatric population? Patient and parent/guardian education is essential with time taken to clearly explain treatment type, usage and rational as well as address concerns. A written action plan (WAP) is extremely helpful [19]. It is important to reassure the child that they are not unique in having this condition and that the treatment they are receiving is used by lots of other children of their age group.

Simple reward measures such as sticker charts may be helpful in younger children, but as they get older, handing greater responsibility to the child for their own care may be more successful.

Ou et al. [16] summarised issues and solutions in childhood adherence as outlined below.

Common reasons for poor adherence and strategies for improvement in different paediatric age groups [16]

Age group	Reasons for poor adherence	Strategies for improvement
Infants	Fear of adverse effects	Choose safe treatments
	Caregiver availability	Emphasise treatment safety
	General beliefs about medication	Schedule return visit shortly after starting treatment to reinforce and re-educate
Young children	Burden of treatment (chasing kids down, time to apply)	Short time between first and follow-up clinic appointments
		Easy-to-use treatment
		Positive reinforcement (e.g. stickers)
Teens	Not wanting to be different/wanting to be like peers	Tell them they are using same products as other teens
	Desire for independence/oppositional behaviour	Give them independence and responsibility for their treatment

3.4.2   Treatment Adherence in Patients with Psoriasis

In 2013, a group from the Dermatology Research Centre at Manchester University [3] performed a systematic literature review looking specifically at medication adherence in patients with psoriasis. This was an electronic search using the terms adherence/compliance/self-management/concordance and psoriasis. Although the initial search resulted in 982 titles, only 29 studies were included once inclusion criteria were applied. The inclusion criteria involved assessing each study's methodological quality by considering generalisability (including sample size), measurement of disease outcome and adherence (direct measures, patient self-report measures, pharmacy prescription refill records, medication weight or number and MEMS – Medication Event Monitoring System) and the data collection and statistical analysis. These studies were critically appraised to answer two questions: What is the extent of non-adherence in psoriasis patients and what factors are associated with non-adherence in this group?

There were then eight determinants that were examined:

1. Sociodemographical factors
2. Disease severity
3. Treatment modality
4. Lifestyle factors
5. Quality of life
6. Psychological distress
7. Patient satisfaction with treatment and consultation
8. Patient-expressed reasons for non-adherence

The overall adherence rate across these studies was variable (14–75 %) but always suboptimal, and some patients showed variation in their own adherence reflecting change in motivation, disease severity or perhaps the "white coat phenomenon" (better adherence on approach to clinic appointment). Looking at each determinant, in turn there were inconsistencies in results. Sociodemography and disease severity did not reliably predict adherence. In the four studies looking at lifestyle factors, one reported lower adherence in those with greater alcohol consumption, and two studies showed lower adherence in smokers. Interestingly, adherence was found to be lower in those who undertake regular physical activity compared to those who lead a more sedentary lifestyle. Although there were no statements within these studies as to why that might be the case, one can postulate theories. In people who are active, they may feel that they don't have time to use their treatment as directed, or it may interfere directly with their ability to carry out said activities. It is possible that people with more severe psoriasis (who may also have psoriatic arthritis) may then become more sedentary. If their psoriasis is more severe, then they maybe on treatment that, although more significant, is easier to adhere to. The two factors that seemed to be most important in predicting adherence were the negative effect of psychological distress and the positive effect of patient satisfaction with their consultation and confidence in the treatment plan. These two latter points must be taken on board by the health-care provider as reassuring the patient addressing concerns and deciding on a treatment plan together is at the heart of adherence and taking time at consultation to discuss these issues is essential to improve adherence rates. Unsurprisingly, these studies also showed that higher adherence is associated with an improvement in disease severity.

3.4.3 Non-adherence in Acne

Although adherence figures vary widely for acne treatment, both oral and topical, it is estimated that adherence rates are around 50% (range reported 7–98%) [5, 20]. This is a rather disappointing figure, especially when one considers the number of consultations that patients may have for this condition and the cost of prescribing multiple treatments that then go unused.

In 2013, Snyder et al. performed a systematic review of studies looking at acne treatment adherence and found an overall adherence rate of oral acne treatment that was 76.3% and, for topical therapy, 75.8% [21]. Better adherence was associated with the following:

- Good understanding of acne and treatment [6]
- More severe acne at outset of treatment
- Single-agent therapy
- Satisfaction with treatment [5]
- Shorter duration of treatment [9]
- Negative impact of acne on quality of life [7, 10]

Risk factors for non-adherence were young age and side effects in more than half of the studies analysed. Forgetfulness also seemed a common reason for reduced adherence. Other factors leading to a reduction in adherence were:

- Treatment dissatisfaction
- Moderate to high DLQI score (i.e. little effect on quality of life by acne)
- Previous systemic therapy
- Lack of symptom improvement
- Lack of treatment knowledge
- Male gender
- Low IQ
- Living alone/single
- Unemployment
- Busy job/social life
- Frustration with treatment
- Comorbidities [5–11]

3.5 Conclusion: Addressing Problems and Finding Solutions

Although there are many other common skin diseases, the pattern is the same for adherence and non-adherence. This pattern may strike some health-care providers as obvious or something they would instinctively recognise. However, hopefully this will highlight the kind of patient that should be considered for more in-depth counselling and make the health-care provider consider management in a more individualised and holistic way.

This final section is a suggestion to the health-care provider of how best to approach the consultation to optimise adherence.

It is always important to have a good rapport with patients as it leads to greater communication and trust. Try to know the patient and understand how their disease affects them in terms of symptoms, relationships, occupation and hobbies. Know what other health issues they have and what medication they take and what sort of burden these have on their day-to-day life. It is helpful to know about the home situation. Who is there? What issues do they have? Are they dependant on the patient? Also try to ascertain what they know of their condition and what their beliefs are in terms of the disease, treatments and prognosis prior to bombarding them with information. Try to address each thing separately and in a language that they understand, and reassure them they are not "the only one". In gathering information about who your patient is outside of your consulting room, you should be in a better position to discuss treatments that will be more suited to that individual.

Taking time to assess and then patiently discuss diagnosis and treatment options with the patient will improve their adherence. Unfortunately, there are often time constraints because of appointment duration, clinics running behind and volume of patients to be seen. If time really is an issue, then give the patient written information, and offer them an appointment in the near future to return and discuss. Another option is to pass them over to another member of the team (e.g. dermatology nurse) for specific education. Providing written information including that of support groups can be very useful, but make sure the patient is literate and that it is in their language.

In terms of treatment, in general the health-care provider should try to keep a regime as simple as possible. This should involve using the least amount of medications and as few applications or administrations per day as possible. For dry skin complaints, the greasiest formulation that the patient will tolerate should be prescribed. In some, this may be liquid paraffin and in others a water-based lotion. If possible, topical therapy should not be staining or malodorous or so thick that it remains visible for a long period of time. Treatments should be easy and quick to apply particularly for morning use and in those who have busy home and work lives.

If oral therapy is given, then ideally once-a-day preparations are better in terms of compliance. If side effects are encountered, then advising patients about these in advance and telling them there are things that can help will encourage them to continue as long as it is safe to do so. If cutaneous side effects are suspected, then topical therapy can be given at the time of initial prescription (e.g. moisturiser samples for patients receiving retinoids).

It is very helpful if patients are able to access someone for advice easily, be it primary or secondary care. Early advice may encourage them to continue with their treatment if a problem is encountered and will reduce prolonged gaps in treatment. Also their confidence in their treatment and the prescriber will be greater. Addressing any problems as they arise will hopefully increase adherence.

Listen to patients, educate them, support them and prescribe treatment for them as individuals.

References

1. World Health Organisation (2003) Adherence to long-term therapies: evidence for action. ISBN 92-4-154599-2
2. National Institute for Health and Clinical Excellence. 3 Mar 2008. Medicines concordance (involving patients in decisions about prescribed medicines) http://www.nice.org.uk/guidance/cg76
3. Thorneloe RJ, Bundy C, Griffiths CEM, Ashcroft DM, Cordingley L (2013) Adherence to medication in patients with psoriasis: a systematic literature review. Br J Dermatol 168(1):20–31
4. Williams J, Clemens S, Olienikova K, Tarvin K (2003) The skills for life survey. A national needs and impact survey of literacy, numeracy and ICT skills. Department for Education and Skills, London
5. Dréno B, Thiboutot D, Gollnick H, Finlay AT, Layton A, Leyden JJ, Leutenegger E, Perez M (2010) Large-scale worldwide observational study of adherence with acne therapy. Int J Dermatol 49(4):448–456

6. Miyachi Y, Hayashi N, Furukawa F, Akamatsu H, Matsunaga K, Watanabe S, Kawashima M (2011) Acne management in Japan: study of patient adherence. Dermatology (Basel, Switzerland) 223(2):174–181
7. Tan JK, Balagurusamy M, Fung K et al (2009) Effect of quality of life impact and clinical severity on adherence to topical acne treatment. J Cutan Med Surg 13:204–208
8. Jones-Caballero M, Pedrosa E, Peñas PF (2008) Self-reported adherence to treatment and quality of life in mild to moderate acne. Dermatology (Basel, Switzerland) 217(4):309–314
9. Mufleh L, Gonzalez M, Judodihardjo H, Finlay AH (1999) Compliance is high in patients taking oral isotretinoin for acne. Br J Dermatol 55(141):87
10. Zaghloul SS, Cunliffe WJ, Goodfield MJ (2005) Objective assessment of compliance with treatments in acne. Br J Dermatol 152(5):1015–1021
11. Tan X, Al-Dabagh A, Davis SA, Lin HC, Balkrishnan R, Chang J, Feldman SR (2013) Medication adherence, healthcare costs and utilization associated with acne drugs in the Medicaid enrolees with acne vulgaris. Am J Clin Dermatol 14(3):243–251
12. Gellad WF, Grenard JL, Marcum ZA (2011) A systematic review of barriers to medication adherence in the elderly: looking beyond cost and regimen complexity. Am J Geriatr Pharmacother 9(1):11–23
13. Koch S, Salem W, Levender MM, Feldman SR (2012) Review of the effect of race/ethnicity on medication adherence. J Am Acad Dermatol 66(4):AB61
14. Sandoval LF, Feldman SR (2013) Biologics in practice: adherence to biologic therapy in psoriasis. Dermatologist 21(2): 30–34
15. Burkhart PV, Dunbar-Jacob J (2002) Adherence research in the paediatric and adolescent populations: a decade in review. In: Hayman L, Mahon MM, Turner JR (eds) Chronic illness in children: an evidence-based approach. Springer, New York
16. Ou HT, Feldman SR, Balkrishnan R (2010) Understanding and improving treatment adherence in paediatric patients. Semin Cutan Med Surg 29:137–140, Elsevier Inc
17. Drotar D, Bonner MS (2009) Influences on adherence to paediatric asthma treatment: a review of correlates and predictors. J Dev Behav Pediatr 30:574–582
18. McQuaid EL, Kopel SJ, Klein RB et al (1992) Medication adherence in pediatric asthma: reasoning, responsibility, and behaviour. J Pediatr Psychol 11:190–198
19. Chisolm SS, Taylor SL, Balkrishnan R et al (2008) Written action plans: potential for improving outcomes in children with atopic dermatitis. J Am Acad Dermatol 59:677–683
20. Ellis RM, Koch LH, McGuire E, Williams JV (2011) Potential barriers to adherence in pediatric dermatology. Pediatr Dermatol 28(3):242–244
21. Snyder S, Crandell I, Davis SA, Feldman SR (2014) Medical adherence to acne therapy: a systematic review. Am J Clin Dermatol 15(2):87–94
22. Shea B, Swindon MV, Tanjong Ghogomu E, Orliz Z, Katchamart W, Rader T, Bombadier C, Wells GA, Tugwell P (2013) Folic acid and folinic acid for reducing side effects in patients receiving methotrexate for rheumatoid arthritis. Cochrane Database Syst Rev (5):CD000951

Chapter 4
Non-attendance, Predictors and Interventions

Katrina Hutton Carlsen, Karen Marie Carlsen, and Jørgen Serup

4.1 Introduction

Adherence is, in dermatology as in other fields, of the uppermost importance for treatment outcome and patient satisfaction, which subsequently will impact quality of life. Non-adherence has been described as a worldwide problem with wide ranging factors. In other chapters of this book, adherence and non-adherence are described in different dermatological patient groups.

Another element closely related to adherence and non-adherence is the complex problem of non-attendance, which is resource consuming and should also be considered a major violation of adherence to treatment. Non-attendance is an obvious topic for study.

Do dermatological patients attend their consultations? If not, for what reasons and who is responsible? What interventions can reduce non-attendance?

These questions have been sought answered, since non-attendance may influence adherence to treatment and, hereby, the overall patient-physician relationship and treatment outcome. To reduce non-adherence, interventions such as early follow-up have been suggested; however, long waiting times for dermatological consultations are an increasing problem. There is an urgent need to focus on non-attendance to ensure that all consultation times are occupied, which will conceivably affect the adherence level in a positive way.

K. Hutton Carlsen • J. Serup (✉)
Department of Dermatology, Bispebjerg University Hospital, Copenhagen, Denmark
e-mail: Katrinahuttoncarlsen@hotmail.com; joergen.vedelskov.serup@regionh.dk

K.M. Carlsen
Centre for Rheumatology, Rigshospitalet, Copenhagen University Hospital,
Copenhagen, Denmark

© Springer International Publishing Switzerland 2016   29
S.A. Davis (ed.), *Adherence in Dermatology*,
DOI 10.1007/978-3-319-30994-1_4

4.2   The Concept "Non-attendance"

Non-attendance is the act of patients failing to attend their planned consultations and, in advance, failing to inform the hospital/clinic department involved.
    Related problems:

- Long waiting lists.
- The non-attendant occupies a consultation another patient could have attended and benefitted from.
- Non-attendance may influence adherence to medication since early follow-up consultations are important for the adjustment of treatment relative to development of disease.
- Impact on quality of life.
- Non-attendance is an economic and practical burden in healthcare and an abuse of resources.

4.3   Non-attendance in the Dermatological Field

Non-attendance (NA) rates and the reasons have been granted little attention in the field of dermatology. Earlier studies from university dermatology clinics reveal a high NA rate; in 1999, an NA rate of 17 % was presented and another study from 2002 showed an NA rate of 21.9 % [1, 2].
    In an Italian survey from 2008, all patients who showed non-attendance at a dermatological clinic were contacted by telephone to determine the reasons. The NA rate was 11.19 % with the main reasons being forgetfulness, work-related problems and concomitant illness [3].
    In a comparable survey from Denmark, NA patients were also contacted by telephone immediately after a missed consultation. Four hundred sixty-nine of 3592 booked patients showed NA (13 %). Main reasons for NA were forgetfulness (34.3 %) and erroneous scheduling (27.7 %); see Fig. 4.1 [4].
    These studies indicate that NA rates during the past years have decreased, presumably due to more focus on efficiency.

4.3.1   Non-attendants

Comparison of age group offenders revealed that children and youngsters from 0 to 25 years showed a higher NA than others [4, 5]. Gender and dermatological conditions had no significant influence on NA [1, 4].
    New patients presented higher NA than patients who were regular visitors to dermatological clinics. In a study of 52,604 consecutive first-time patients, the NA rate was 27.6 % [3]. This rate is very high compared to 17.1 %, 19 % and 20 % found

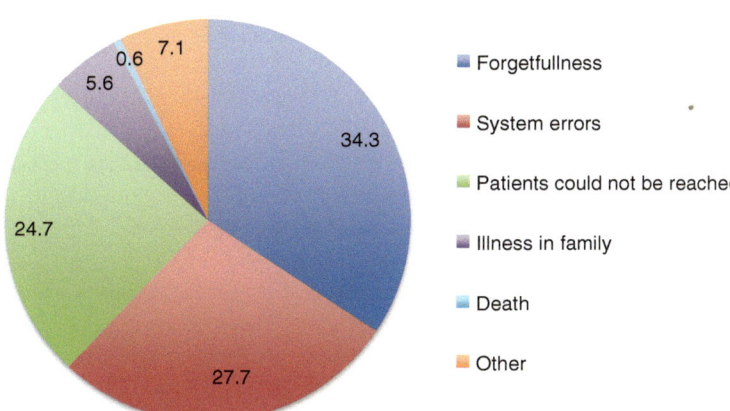

Fig. 4.1 Reasons for non-attendance (NA) in a dermatology clinic in Denmark

in other studies [4, 6, 7]. However, it can be concluded from all studies that first-time patients present higher NA than others.

Forgetfulness has been reported in 23–25 % of new referrals [6, 7] and NA due to "skin condition already improved" in 46 % [7]. However, patients are not responsible for the whole problem. Inadequate communication between the hospital/clinic and patients has also been reported as a reason for NA (17 % and 27.7 %) with erroneous scheduling (Fig. 4.2): no information/letter supplied with details of appointment, failure of handicap transportation (which in Denmark is the hospital's responsibility) and overloaded hospital telephone lines [4, 6]. Hospitals are also accountable for the high NA rates and should therefore endeavour to reduce them.

4.4   Suggestions for Improving Attendance

In the following, suggestions for improving attendance will be presented. Multiple suggestions have been drafted in the literature, some more adequate than others.

4.4.1   *Payments and Fines*

Comparisons between state-subsidised dermatology departments and private clinics where patients determine their own appointments reveal that NA rates are higher in state-subsidised departments, exemplified with NA rates of 26 % compared to 13 % and 7.79 % in private clinics and insurance programmes [1, 8]. Here it should be

System error types in percentage

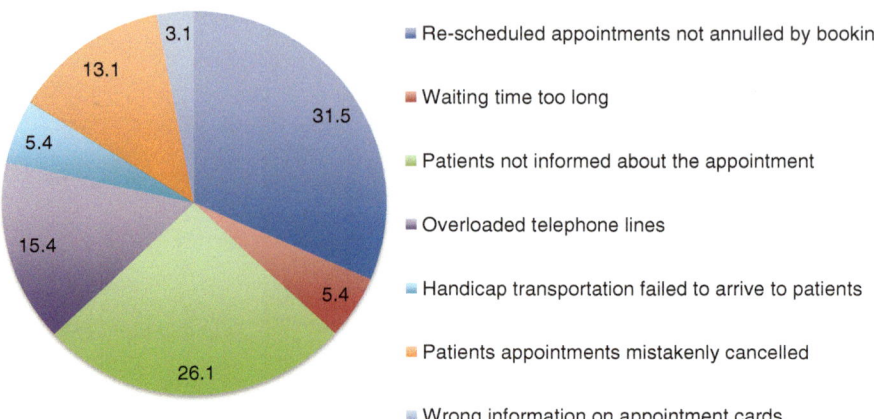

Fig. 4.2 System errors were reported in 130 cases of 469 non-attendant patients (27.7%) in a dermatology clinic in Denmark. The following system errors were attributed

mentioned that in many private clinics, fines are administered for failing to comply with an appointment.

However, newer studies gathered from different countries have shown that NA rates in state-subsidised dermatology departments have improved [3, 4], indicating that more focus on the problem of NA has had a positive effect.

4.4.2   "Final Warning" Letters and Life-Long Exclusions from Clinics

It has been suggested that patients repeatedly showing non-attendance should receive a "warning" letter explaining the consequences of further occurrences of NA, i.e. termination of further treatment. Awareness of multiple non-attendances in a dermatology department led to a reduction of further consultations to NA patients from 74 to 50.4% [4]. However, patients with serious diseases should not have their treatments terminated.

Life-long exclusions from clinics should not be an option. As illustrated, the reasons for non-attendance are numerous, and patients, hospitals and clinics can all contribute to improve NA rates. Focus should not be on who is the cause, but on methods to improve NA rates. Dermatological patients are burdened by their skin diseases and should have the possibility of receiving help. However, at university state-subsidised dermatology departments, where no fines are administered, patients who continuously fail to comply should be referred back to their GP for follow-up and those admitting NA was due to improved dermatological status should have their ongoing treatment at the department terminated.

4.4.3 SMS Notification

SMS notification has proved to be an efficient and inexpensive method to improve NA rates especially among the younger generation who have the highest NA rates among the different age groups [9]. This improvement is presumably because this generation possess more mobile telephones (smartphones), capable of receiving SMS messages, than the elder groups and is more apt at using them [3, 9]. In general, the majority have a positive opinion of SMS reminders, albeit a mere 17.7 % had enrolled in the notification system, while 33 % were unaware of it. Automatic enrolment when referring patients would improve these results [9]. It is a prerequisite; all health professionals and patients ensure updated contact details.

E-mail notification is also an option although there is a risk of reminders ending as spam mails and therefore lost. Another aspect is that not all patients read their e-mails regularly.

4.4.4 Appointments Made on the Internet

Appointments made online are in all likelihood to have lower non-attendance rates than appointments made through traditional means. A study analysing appointment records from three dermatology clinics located outside of Houston, Texas, USA, which were planned over the Internet, revealed a non-attendance rate of 6.9 % [10]. Telephone lines at dermatology departments are often overloaded making cancellations difficult to accomplish [4, 11]. Possible solutions could be opening more telephone lines or installing an answering machine although the latter could result in no new appointment for the patient.

E-medicine and Internet communication with dermatologists have a number of limitations, which could result in diagnostic misconception and also give rise to medication errors.

4.4.5 Shorter Waiting Time and Early Follow-Up Visits

Longer waiting time has an influence on both NA and adherence to treatment [12, 13]. Either overbooking dermatologists' daily schedules or a more consequent position towards continuous NA offenders could reduce waiting lists. In a deliberately overbooked schedule, a non-attendant would not have an influence on the productivity of a department or clinic.

A study of an intervention programme designed to reduce waiting times for dermatological appointments showed a decrease from 29.3 to 6.8 days by means of patient overbooking and centralisation of the service [14]. The number of scheduled appointments over a 6-month period rose from 17,007 to 20,433. However, a negative consequence of overbooking, which should be taken into consideration, could be a stressful working atmosphere for medical staff.

4.4.6 Clear and Accurate Information Concerning Consultations

Correct appointment details on appointment cards with information on date, weekday, time and location should be accurate and clear. In dermatology, erroneous details on appointment cards have been reported in 3.1 %. It is a small percentage but, nevertheless, should be improved [4].

Patients receiving oral information should repeat information to reduce the risk of errors.

Letters with appointments should arrive timely allowing the patient to make arrangements to attend consultation or to cancel the appointment.

Patients should be informed about the importance of attending consultations and cancellations both for their own health and for patients who could have the opportunity of attending instead.

4.5 Conclusions

Non-attendance (NA) is a major economic waste for the healthcare system and creates an unused capacity leading to longer waiting lists. Although NA rates appear to have fallen during the past years, non-attendance remains a problem. Factors influencing NA can vary from clinic to clinic and should therefore be examined individually. Progress requires analysis of the precise problem in a specific clinic or hospital followed by multidisciplinary undertakings involving patients, secretaries and medical staff. Everybody has a responsibility in reducing NA. Online bookings, correct appointment details on appointment cards and SMS reminders are some actions to improve appointment attendance.

References

1. Penneys NS, Glaser DA (1999) The incidence of cancellation and non-attendance at a dermatology clinic. J Am Acad Dermatol 40:714–718
2. Canizares MJ, Penneys NS (2002) The incidence of nonattendance at an urgent care dermatology clinic. J Am Acad Dermatol 46:457–459
3. Cusini M, Auxilia F, Trevisan V, Visconti U, Castaldi S (2008) A telephone survey on the reasons for non-attendance in a dermatological clinic. G Ital Dermatol Venereol 143:353–357

4. Carlsen KH, Carlsen KM, Serup J (2011) Non-attendance rate in a Danish University Clinic of Dermatology. J Eur Acad Dermatol Venereol 25:1269–1274
5. Cohen AD, Dreiher J, Vardy DA, Weitzman D (2008) Nonattendance in a dermatology clinic – a large sample analysis. J Eur Acad Dermatol Venereol 22:1178–1183
6. Bottomley WW, Cotterill JA (1994) An audit of the factors involved in new patient non-attendance in a dermatology out-patient department. Clin Exp Dermatol 19:399–400
7. Hon KL, Leung TF, Wong Y, Ma KC, Fok TF (2005) Reasons for new referral non-attendance at a pediatric dermatology center: a telephone survey. J Dermatol Treat 16:113–116
8. Pehr K (2007) No show: incidence of nonattendance at a dermatology practice in a single universal payer model. J Cutan Med Surg 11:53–56
9. Carlsen KH, Eliasen TU, Carlsen KM, Serup J (2014) SMS reminders can reduce non-attendance at consultations. Ugeskr Laeger 176(38). pii: V03140176
10. Siddiqui Z, Rashid R (2013) Cancellations and patient access to physicians: ZocDoc and the evolution of e-medicine. Dermatol Online J 19:14
11. Verbov J (1992) Why 100 patients failed to keep an outpatient appointment-audit in a dermatology department. J R Soc Med 85:277–278
12. Cohen AD, Goldbart AD, Levi I, Shapiro J, Vardy DA (2007) Health provider factors associated with nonattendance in pediatric dermatology ambulatory patients. Pediatr Dermatol 24:113–117
13. Davis SA, Lin HC, Yu CH, Balkrishnan R, Feldman SR (2014) Underuse of early follow-up visits: a missed opportunity to improve patients' adherence. J Drugs Dermatol 13:833–836
14. Bibi Y, Cohen AD, Goldfarb D, Rubinshtein E, Vardy DA (2007) Intervention program to reduce waiting time of a dermatological visit: managed overbooking and service centralization as effective management tools. Int J Dermatol 46:830–834

Part II
Methods of Measuring Adherence

Chapter 5
Using Retrospective Databases to Study Adherence

Scott A. Davis and Steven R. Feldman

Retrospective analyses of claims databases are one of the most common tools to study real-world adherence patterns. These analyses are frequently used to determine adherence rates within specific populations [1, 2], compare adherence across multiple diseases or medications [3], or investigate how adherence changes over time [4, 5]. Investigating changes over time can include patient-level analyses showing trends in how many patients are still adherent or persistent at a certain number of months after initiating treatment [4]. A very different example of tracking adherence over time would use calendar time rather than time from each individual patient's initiation of treatment, such as for assessing the impact of a policy change on adherence. For example, a policymaker may want to know if a reduction in co-payments for a medication led to improved adherence [5].

This chapter will begin by explaining reasons why retrospective database studies can provide information that is difficult or impossible to obtain from prospective randomized designs. Next, a step-by-step guide for formulating a research question, choosing a study population and database, and quantifying adherence will be presented. Methods for calculating the two most common adherence outcome measures, Medication Possession Ratio and Percentage of Days Covered, will be explained. Finally, details of specific study designs will be presented, and a few limitations of database methodologies will be discussed.

S.A. Davis (✉)
Department of Dermatology, Wake Forest School of Medicine, Winston-Salem, NC, USA

Division of Pharmaceutical Outcomes and Policy, University of North Carolina Eshelman School of Pharmacy, Chapel Hill, NC, USA
e-mail: sdavis81@email.unc.edu

S.R. Feldman
Departments of Dermatology, Pathology, and Public Health Sciences, Wake Forest School of Medicine, Winston-Salem, NC, USA

© Springer International Publishing Switzerland 2016
S.A. Davis (ed.), *Adherence in Dermatology*,
DOI 10.1007/978-3-319-30994-1_5

5.1   Why Do We Need Retrospective Database Studies?

The traditional prejudice against nonrandomized designs in the health sciences is still strong, but there are many reasons that observational studies are needed to complement randomized controlled trials (RCTs). First, claims databases often provide sample sizes that are as much as two or three orders of magnitude greater than large RCTs. Second, RCTs are also limited in time, often ranging from a few weeks up to 1 year. For research questions investigating long-term outcomes, data sources that can follow patients over longer periods of time are needed. Third, RCTs often have very restrictive inclusion/exclusion criteria that exclude specific populations that may be of interest. RCTs often exclude the elderly, children, pregnant women, people with certain comorbidities or concomitant medications, or other groups in which there may be a heightened concern about medication safety. RCTs are normally restricted to people who are willing and able to volunteer for the study and may introduce Hawthorne effects in which study subjects behave differently because they are being observed. On the other hand, retrospective studies can investigate how typical real-world patients behave when they are not being actively observed or given extra office visits, as most clinical trial protocols require. Finally, there are some research questions for which it is unethical or impossible to randomize subjects. For example, it is unethical to randomize patients to a placebo when there is a known effective treatment available. Adherence (as a cause of clinical outcomes) is another example, since it is impossible to randomize patients to take or not take their medication as directed. (Adherence as an outcome in trials will be discussed in the next chapter.)

The main limitation to nonrandomized designs is the potential for bias due to systematic differences between groups, which are eliminated in expectation[1] by the process of randomization. Fortunately, epidemiologists have developed many methods for limiting bias and ensuring comparable groups. These methods include stratification, restriction, matching, adjustment for covariates in regression models, and a variety of propensity score methods. A full discussion of such methods is beyond the scope of this book, but can be found in standard pharmacoepidemiology textbooks [6].

---

[1] That is, as the sample size gets larger, the probability of a substantial difference between the groups decreases until it is highly unlikely (P value very close to zero) with very large samples.

5.2   Step-by-Step Guide to Study Design and Analysis

5.2.1   Formulating the Research Question

There are a variety of different motivations for performing a retrospective adherence study in dermatology. Nolan and Feldman's article "Adherence, the Fourth Dimension in the Geometry of Dermatological Treatment" suggests a framework for thinking about how to ask these questions [7]. For example, one might observe that a medication does not seem to work as well in everyday practice as it does in clinical trials. A treatment may initially work well, but then seem to decline in effectiveness over time. A treatment might seem not to work very well in a certain demographic or cultural group, even though it works in other groups. Maybe we even see that a lower (0.5 %) concentration of topical 5-fluorouracil for actinic keratoses strangely seems to work better than a higher concentration [8]. These phenomena may give rise to hypotheses we can test in databases. We might hypothesize that patients have low adherence to the medication that does not work outside of clinical trials. We might test whether the treatment that loses effectiveness over time is subject to declining adherence over time. If a treatment does not work in particular demographic or cultural groups, we might see whether those groups have lower adherence. We might hypothesize that the 0.5 % 5-fluorouracil works better because patients actually use it, whereas the 5 % formulation is too irritating to keep taking. To explore whether adherence explains the observed results, patients' adherence can be measured in a database and plotted over time, or compared across different groups. If adherence is low, the results suggest a need for interventions or changes in practice to help patients use the medications better.

If an intervention to improve adherence has already been undertaken, such as a new policy to improve access to a drug, then a database study with a pre-post design may be helpful to determine whether the policy worked. On the other hand, some policies may have unintended negative effects on adherence, such as black box warnings or new prior authorization requirements. The event does not even need to be a policy; it could be a celebrity endorsing a specific medication or the publication of a study suggesting a medication is unsafe. Whether the expected effect is positive or negative, and regardless of what caused the event, the same pre-post design with segmented regression (discussed in Sect. 5.2.4 below) can be used to test the hypothesis that there was a change in adherence [9].

5.2.2   Choosing a Study Population and Data Source

In the USA, the most common claims data are aggregated from large health plans, such as the UnitedHealth database, or multiple insurance plans, such as in the Truven MarketScan® Commercial, Medicare, and Medicaid databases [10, 11]. Medicare data are excellent for studying diseases affecting mainly older populations ages 65 and older, while commercial or Medicaid data are suitable for diseases affecting all ages [10]. Medicaid data have the benefit of a more stable enrollment, since enrollees tend to stay in Medicaid longer than in any particular private insurance plan. However, results from Medicaid data will generally be generalizable only to populations of similar socioeconomic status.

Many other countries have outstanding national databases intended to capture all prescriptions dispensed within the country, such as Denmark, Norway, Sweden, and the Netherlands [10]. In the United Kingdom, the clinical practice research database is based on a representative sample of medical records from practitioners in the National Health Service (NHS). Canada also has an excellent system of healthcare databases, but each province maintains a separate database [10]. In general, the best national databases have significant advantages over those used in the USA. In a national health system, patients typically never disenroll from the national health plan unless they emigrate, so they can be followed for long time periods. Some databases have extensive clinical and lab data that may help to provide additional important patient characteristics, such as disease severity. Most countries use ICD-10 codes rather than ICD-9-CM, which can provide an extra level of detail for some diseases. For example, severe psoriasis has a separate ICD-10 code from mild psoriasis, whereas in the ICD-9-CM system, all psoriasis is coded with a single code. In the absence of a separate code for severe psoriasis, researchers would have to infer the severity of psoriasis from the medications prescribed, which is certainly not ideal in light of the frequent undertreatment of psoriasis. Another benefit is that some databases provide easy linkage to other data sources, such as rare disease registries. Although studies requiring linkage between multiple databases are not necessarily impossible in the USA, the general unwillingness to use a common identifier for a patient across multiple databases greatly impedes the ability to perform these studies in US data.

5.2.3 Quantifying Adherence: Measures of Adherence

Several measures of adherence are commonly used in reporting results from database studies on adherence. The most common are Medication Possession Ratio (MPR) and the newer Percentage of Days Covered (PDC) [12].

The MPR is customarily calculated as the number of total days supply of medication dispensed in the period of interest, divided by the time from first fill to the last fill, plus the number of days supplied at the last fill. For example, if a patient received six 30-day prescriptions for a medication on days 1, 31, 61, 91, 121, and 151 of a 180-day period, MPR would be $(30*6)/((151-1)+30)$ or 100% (Fig. 5.1a). Adding the days supply of the last fill can cause the denominator to include some days that are beyond the last day of available data. Therefore, if the patient received the first prescription on the first day and the sixth prescription on the 180th day, 29 days would need to be added to the denominator, lowering the MPR to $(30*6)/209$ or 86% (Fig. 5.1b). If the patient received the first prescription on the 30th day and the

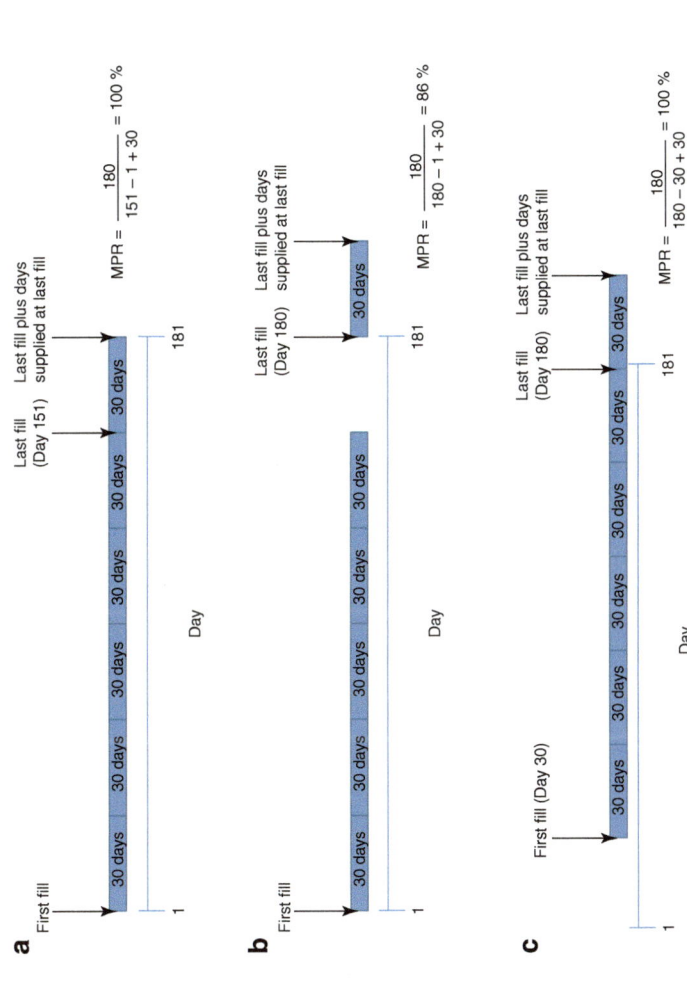

Fig. 5.1 (**a**) MPR calculation for first fill on day 1 and last fill on day 151. (**b**) MPR calculation for first fill on day 1 and last fill on day 180. The period used in the denominator can extend up to the number of days supplied at the last fill past the end of observation time. (**c**) MPR calculation for first fill on day 30 and last fill on day 180. The period used in the denominator now does not begin until day 30 and extends past the end of observation

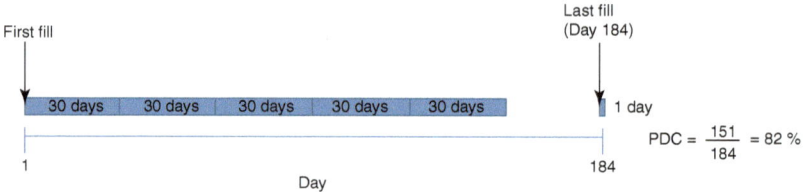

Fig. 5.2 PDC calculation analogous to the MPR calculation in Fig. 5.1b. In this case, the last prescription is truncated at the end of the predefined 6-month period; so despite the patient receiving a 30-day prescription, only 1 day of supply is counted

sixth prescription on the 180th day, then only the days from 30 to 210 would count, and the MPR would still be 180/180 or 100 % (Fig. 5.1c).

The PDC is calculated as the number of total days with medication available, divided by the length of the follow-up period. Often PDC calculations are based on a fixed period of calendar time – say, a 6-month period from May 1, 2015, to October 31, 2015. In this case the length of the follow-up period is the time from the first fill within the year of observation to the end of the period (Fig. 5.2). As with MPR, days preceding the first fill are counted toward neither the numerator nor the denominator. However, with PDC, the last prescription is also truncated at the end of the period, so that a patient who fills a 30-day prescription on the last day of the period (October 31, 2015) is credited with only 1 day of supply for that fill. On the other hand, with MPR, the full 30 days of supply would be counted, and the denominator time would also be extended until 29 days past the last day of the period (i.e., November 29, 2015). Unlike MPR, PDC cannot exceed 100 % since a patient either is or is not covered on a particular day, so the maximum days covered are equal to the length of the follow-up period.

Depending on the research question of interest, the PDC can also be calculated starting on the day of the first fill or diagnosis date and continuing for a fixed length of time.

PDC has been implicitly endorsed by the US Centers for Medicare and Medicaid Services (CMS) through its inclusion in quality measures for Medicare Part D prescription drug plans. A plan can get anywhere from one to five stars based on a list of 18 quality measures related to prescription drug benefits [13]. The Patient Protection and Affordable Care Act (PPACA) gives legal force to this new system by establishing rewards and penalties for plans having high or low star ratings [14]. Five-star plans are given significant advantages, such as the ability to enroll participants outside of the usually scheduled annual window, while plans that persistently get less than three stars can be shut down [15]. At the time of this writing, the rating system only assesses adherence to renin-angiotensin system antagonists, statins, and four classes of oral antidiabetics [16]. However, the use of PDC as a quality measure is growing in all areas of medicine, and CMS is expected to continue expanding its use in ways that may eventually have considerable impact on the evaluation of dermatologic healthcare delivery. Accountable care organizations (ACOs) are also evaluated partly based on their enrollees' adherence. As ACOs

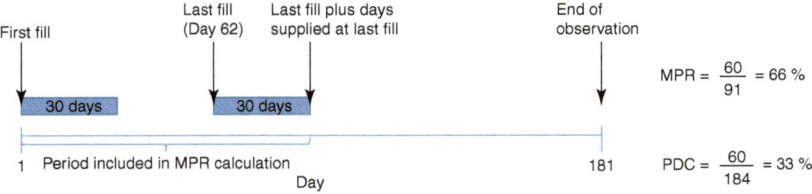

Fig. 5.3 When there is a long period of nonpersistence after the end of the days supplied at the last fill, MPR produces a much higher estimate of adherence than PDC does, since it stops at the end of the days supplied at the last fill

continue to grow, health systems are starting to prepare for a time when they will need to report adherence data from their electronic medical records (EMR) systems to demonstrate their quality of care.

The main difference between MPR and PDC is that the length of the period is typically defined by the first and last fill for MPR, while it is a predetermined follow-up time for PDC (Figs. 5.1, 5.2, and 5.3). The length of the period for MPR is the time between the first and last fill dates, plus the days supplied at the last fill, whereas for PDC, it is either a fixed period of calendar time or a fixed length of time starting at the first fill. The effect is that patients are not penalized for nonpersistence (early discontinuation) when calculating MPR, whereas they are penalized for nonpersistence when calculating PDC. For example, in a study with 6-month follow-up, a patient who filled one 30-day prescription on May 1, 2015, and a second and final 30-day prescription on July 1, 2015, would have an MPR of 60/91 = 66 %, but a PDC of only 60/184 = 33 % (Fig. 5.3). The PDC counts the post-discontinuation period from July 31 to October 31, 2015, as a period of nonadherence, while the MPR ignores it.

Nonetheless, the terminology is not completely standardized, and some studies have referred to their measure as MPR while using a fixed-length study period, truncating adherence at 100 %, or other modifications of the simple MPR [17]. Therefore, it is imperative to read the full methods section of a study reporting adherence using claims data and not assume the authors used a specific methodology based on the name of the measure reported.

5.2.4   Conducting the Study

5.2.4.1   Single-Group Design

The simplest type of retrospective study of adherence may be one that simply seeks to answer the question, "What are the patterns of adherence in patients' prescribed medication X in group Y over time frame Z?" For example, a study might seek to assess patterns of adherence in patients ages 18–64 from a commercially insured US population-prescribed psoriasis medication over a 6-month time frame. This study would use a new-user design [18], requiring patients to have a 6-month wash-out period without any diagnosis of psoriasis preceding the first diagnosis (index date). In the single-group case, it might be acceptable to use a prevalent-user design depending on the research question being asked. The new-user design answers the question, "How do patients use their medication in the first 6 months after their initial prescription for treatment of a certain disease?" A prevalent-user design, on the other hand, would answer the question, "At any point in time, how is the total population with a certain disease using medications for treatment of that disease?"

The single-group design still may contain a subgroup analysis of different populations, in which case the possibility of bias from confounding may still be present. For example, acne patients who use isotretinoin seem to have higher adherence than other acne patients (Chap. 9). However, patients on isotretinoin are a population with higher average disease severity and willingness to navigate the cumbersome iPLEDGE system to get their medication, a source of selection bias. Therefore, the difference in adherence must be interpreted in light of these underlying group differences. If there is interest in removing confounding by acne severity, patients can be matched on acne severity if a measure of acne severity is available in the database. If not, then more advanced methods of dealing with confounding, such as propensity scores [19], might need to be used.

The steps in conducting an adherence study in a single population include:

1. Define the population (by disease state and/or medication) to be studied.
2. Choose the time frame for follow-up. Often it is difficult to determine when the patient was directed to stop medication, so the time frame should be short enough that discontinuation due to successful therapy is not misclassified as nonadherence. However, it should be long enough so that a patient would need multiple medication fills during the period; otherwise patients' adherence would likely be overestimated.
3. Choose the look-back period. Typically patients are required to be continuously enrolled for the duration of the washout period and the follow-up period, such as 6 months before (washout) and after (follow-up) the index date. A longer look-back period reduces the number of patients misclassified as new users who are actually prevalent users and improves ascertainment of covariates [20]. For example, a study in which Charlson Comorbidity Index (CCI) is included as a predictor of adherence would only capture comorbidities if there is a claim for the relevant comorbid diagnosis during the look-back period. On the other hand, a longer look-back period also generally requires exclusion of patients who were not continuously enrolled in the health plan for the entire look-back period. Since the average enrollment time of US commercially insured patients in a single health plan is only 2.5 years, a significant loss of sample size may occur, and selection bias in favor of patients who rarely change health plans can be introduced.
4. Choose the measure of adherence to be used, such as MPR or PDC, and determine which medications will be counted toward the calculation of the measure. These may be all medications indicated for the disease according to accepted practice guidelines. In claims data, it is not generally possible to determine the

exact disease that a medication is prescribed for, such as antibiotics that are prescribed for dermatological and non-dermatological conditions. If there is a great deal of uncertainty, sensitivity analysis with and without inclusion of the problematic medications may help to determine lower and upper bounds on the adherence outcome.

5. Create the cohort. In a relational claims database in which enrollee information and prescription drug claims are in separate tables, such as Truven MarketScan®, this step will involve creating a cohort of those continuously enrolled for the period of interest and having the relevant diagnosis, then joining it to a table of pharmacy claims to obtain all medication fills for the eligible patients. These data can then be limited to those fills that occur within the follow-up period and are for clinically relevant medications.

6. Calculate the adherence measure. A publicly available SAS macro can be used for calculating PDC [21].

7. Perform any additional analyses desired, such as multiple regression to identify significant predictors of adherence, or t tests to compare adherence between subgroups. To assess predictors of adherence, logistic regression is often preferred, requiring the MPR or PDC to be dichotomized at some cutoff. Often 80 % is used as a customary but rather arbitrary cutoff, although it is better to decide the cutoff based on specific clinical knowledge about the forgiveness of the medication. Linear regression can also be used if continuous adherence is considered a more accurate measure of patient behavior. In that case, the assumptions of linear regression (existence, independence, linearity, homoscedasticity, and normal distribution) should be checked to make sure the model is a good fit [22].

5.2.4.2 Comparative Design

In a comparative design, two or more cohorts are selected, such as users of oral vs. topical medications for acne. Since analyses of claims data do not use randomization – the treatment is chosen by the patient and provider, not by the investigator – baseline characteristics of the cohorts may be different, so interpretation of the results must be made carefully. If the two cohorts contain patients prescribed drugs from the same class, such as two different branded topical retinoids, then the results are more likely to be comparable. Despite inevitable barriers to interpreting any observed difference as a causal effect, determining the differences in adherence among patients prescribed different medications is still useful as an exploratory analysis. Such data can then be used to inform efforts to improve adherence in populations prescribed specific medications associated with especially low adherence.

For a comparative new-user design, ideally patients who receive any of the classes of medications under consideration during the washout period would be excluded from all cohorts [23]. For example, if the study is to compare adherence to biologics vs. methotrexate for psoriasis, patients prescribed with either biologics or methotrexate during the washout period would be excluded. However, if it is typical to start with one treatment and then augment with the other treatment, an overwhelming proportion of patients in one cohort might be lost. In a health system where patients are required to fail methotrexate therapy before they may try biologics, disallowing any methotrexate prescription during the washout period might disqualify essentially all biologics patients. There is no perfect solution to this issue, but one possible design would be to compare patients who augment therapy to new users of methotrexate alone.

5.2.4.3 Assessment of Policy Intervention or Event: Pre-Post Design

A further design that is commonly used is a pre-post design for studying the impact of an event, such as a policy intervention, on adherence [9, 24]. In this situation, adherence is calculated for each of several time periods before and after the event, and line segments are fit to the points before and the points after. A model called segmented regression can be used to include both the time frames before and after the event in a single equation, and test whether the slope and/or the level of the line changed at the time of the event (Fig. 5.4) [9]. To make the design more robust, a control group can be introduced, such as another state that is similar in most respects, except that it did not implement the policy [24]. For example, in the hypothetical data for Fig. 5.5, North Carolina implemented a new policy on January 1, 2011, and saw an increase in adherence, but South Carolina never implemented the policy and still saw a similar increase in adherence. The policy does not look as favorable once the control group is added, suggesting that another event that happened to occur around the time of the policy was more likely the cause of the increase in adherence.

5.2.5 Common Limitations of Claims Database Studies of Adherence

It is usually very difficult to use claims data to assess primary nonadherence, in which patients do not ever fill a prescription. Studies are typically limited to patients who filled at least one prescription medication at some point, since it is not known whether patients with no fills are actually addressing their condition with over-the-counter treatments or lifestyle changes. Fortunately, other types of studies have been done to quantify primary nonadherence, which can be close to 50 % in certain dermatologic conditions such as psoriasis [25].

A claims database is derived from insurer data on what was submitted for reimbursement. Medications that are purchased outside of the insurance system are not likely to be captured [26, 27]. These would include over-the-counter medications, generic medications dispensed outside the insurance system (the so-called $4 generics), and medications considered "lifestyle drugs" and thus not reimbursed by some insurance plans or free samples. The data must also be as complete as possible for

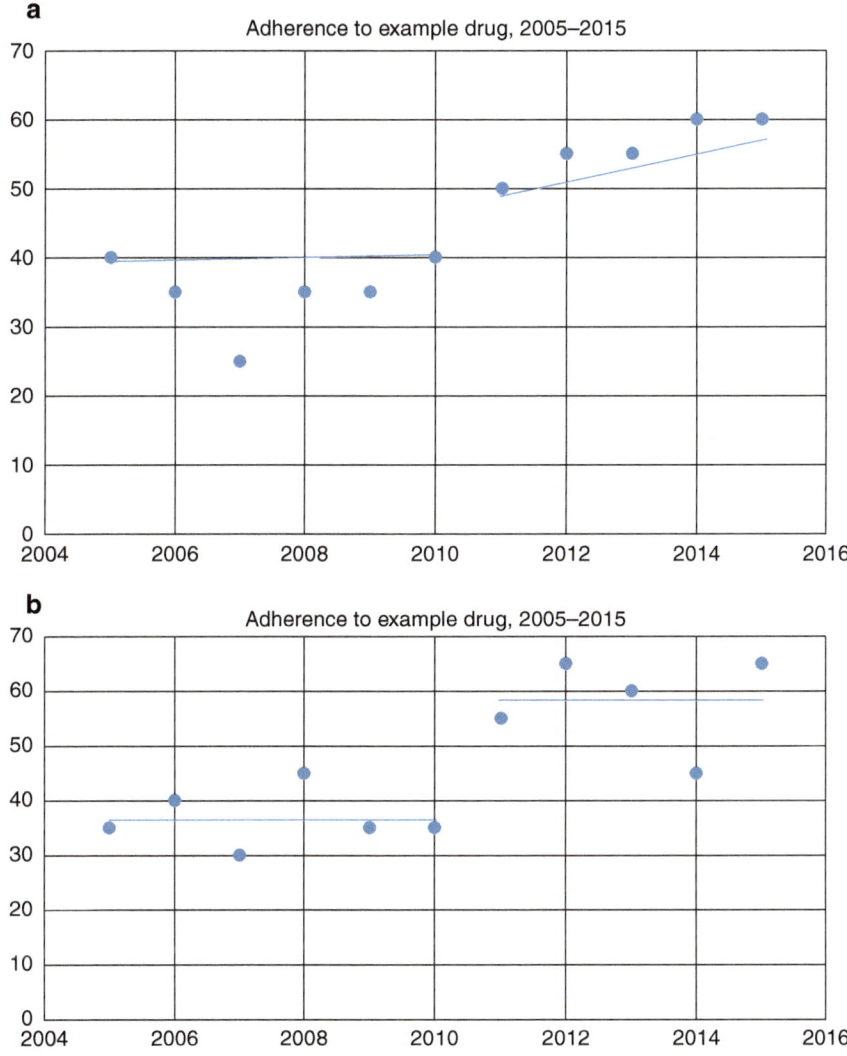

Fig. 5.4 (**a**) Example showing change in both level and slope of the adherence outcome following a new policy that went into place on January 1, 2011. (**b**) Example showing change in level without change in slope of the adherence outcome following a new policy that went into place on January 1, 2011

the population of interest. For example, a study using only Medicare data would generally lack Medicaid claims for dual-eligible patients, so it would have to exclude those patients.

Dermatologic treatment can be especially complex as compared to some other areas of medicine, with frequent medication switches and augmentation or reduction of therapeutic regimens over time [28]. Some patients may use combination regi-

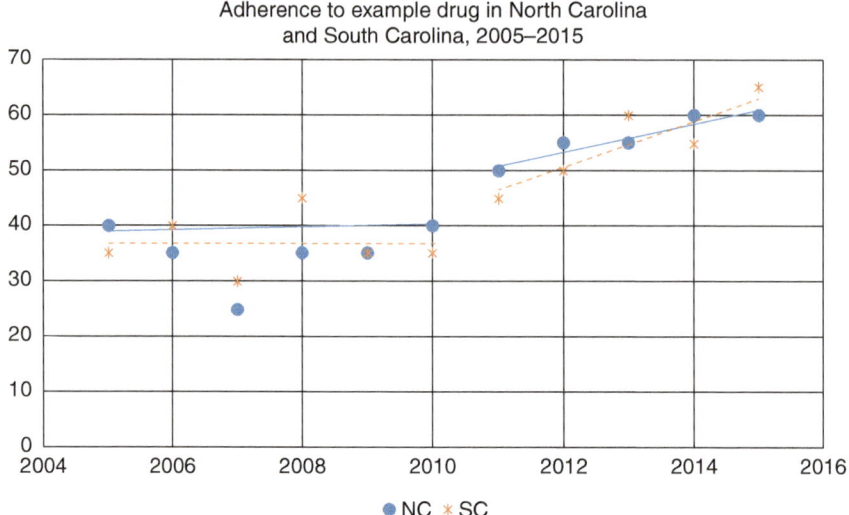

Fig. 5.5 Analysis of adherence to a hypothetical drug in North Carolina (NC) and South Carolina (SC) using segmented regression. The change in both states – one of which implemented a new policy while the other did not – suggests that the policy may not have been the cause of the change

mens, which may consist of combination products, such as adapalene/benzoyl peroxide for acne, or separate products prescribed simultaneously. The management of combination therapies in claims data is not standardized and may depend on the research question. If adherence to a specific drug is the primary interest, then all claims for other drugs might be ignored and patients considered nonadherent if they do not continue to refill the same drug. If general adherence to treatment for a disease is of interest, then all claims for any drug indicated for the disease might be included.

With topical medications, dosing may differ greatly from patient to patient due to varying body surface area of disease, but the days supply given in claims databases may assume a specific, standardized dose. Calculation of PDC using standardized algorithms intended for oral medications may incorrectly estimate the PDC. It may be worth adding a grace period to the end of each patient's days supply to allow for some variation in dosage (Lund JL, 21 Apr 2015, personal communication). For example, with a 15-day grace period, a patient who consistently obtains a 30-day supply of topical medication exactly every 45 days could be considered completely adherent.

Electronic medical records (EMR) data may help overcome some of the limitations of typical claims databases. EMR data may have more specific information on the patient's disease type and severity, as well as dates when patients were advised to discontinue or switch medications. In some integrated delivery systems, it is even becoming possible for physicians to look at their own EMR data to determine which patients are struggling with adherence. These patients can then receive a quick follow-up call to inquire about potential barriers to adherence or other adherence-enhancing interventions discussed in the last section of this book.

References

1. Tan X, Al-Dabagh A, Davis SA et al (2013) Medication adherence, healthcare costs and utilization associated with acne drugs in Medicaid enrollees with acne vulgaris. Am J Clin Dermatol 14(3):243–251
2. Bhosle MJ, Feldman SR, Camacho FT et al (2006) Medication adherence and health care costs associated with biologics in Medicaid-enrolled patients with psoriasis. J Dermatol Treat 17(5):294–301
3. Yeaw J, Benner JS, Walt JG et al (2009) Comparing adherence and persistence across 6 chronic medication classes. J Manag Care Pharm 15(9):728–740
4. Blaschke T, Osterberg L, Vrijens B, Urquhart J (2012) Adherence to medications: insights arising from studies on the unreliable link between prescribed and actual drug dosing histories. Annu Rev Pharmacol Toxicol 52:275–301
5. Maciejewski ML, Wansink D, Lindquist JH et al (2014) Value-based insurance design program in North Carolina increased medication adherence but was not cost neutral. Health Aff (Millwood) 33(2):300–308
6. Schneeweiss S, Suissa S (2013) Advanced approaches to controlling confounding in pharmacoepidemiologic studies. In: Strom BL, Kimmel SE, Hennessy S (eds) Textbook of pharmacoepidemiology. Wiley-Blackwell, Chichester
7. Nolan BV, Feldman SR (2009) Adherence, the fourth dimension in the geometry of dermatological treatment. Arch Dermatol 145(11):1319–1321
8. Hagele TJ, Levender MM, Davis SA et al (2012) Practice trends in the treatment of actinic keratosis in the United States: 0.5% fluorouracil and combination cryotherapy plus fluorouracil are underused despite evidence of benefit. J Cutan Med Surg 16(2):107–114
9. Wagner AK, Soumerai SB, Zhang F, Ross-Degnan D (2002) Segmented regression analysis of interrupted time series studies in medication use research. J Clin Pharm Ther 27(4):299–309
10. Toh S, Andrade SE, Raebel MA et al (2013) Examples of existing automated databases. In: Strom BL, Kimmel SE, Hennessy S (eds) Textbook of pharmacoepidemiology. Wiley-Blackwell, Chichester
11. Quint JB (2015) Health research data for the real world: the MarketScan® databases. Truven Health Analytics, Ann Arbor
12. Nau DP Proportion of days covered (PDC) as a preferred method of measuring adherence. Available at http://www.pqaalliance.org/images/uploads/files/PQA%20PDC%20vs%20%20MPR.pdf. Accessed 29 Dec 2015
13. Young GJ, Rickles NM, Chou CH, Raver E (2014) Socioeconomic characteristics of enrollees appear to influence performance scores for medicare part D contractors. Health Aff (Millwood) 33(1):140–146
14. American Pharmacists Association and Academy of Managed Care Pharmacy (2014) Medicare star ratings: stakeholder proceedings on community pharmacy and managed care partnerships in quality. J Am Pharm Assoc 54(3):e238–e250
15. Reid RO, Deb P, Howell BL, Shrank WH (2013) Association between Medicare advantage plan star ratings and enrollment. JAMA 309(3):267–274
16. Pharmacy Quality Alliance Executive update on medication quality measures in medicare part D plan ratings 2013. Available at http://pqaalliance.org/measures/cms.asp. Accessed 29 Dec 2015
17. Martin BC, Wiley-Exley EK, Richards S et al (2009) Contrasting measures of adherence with simple drug use, medication switching, and therapeutic duplication. Ann Pharmacother 43(1):36–44
18. Ray WA (2003) Evaluating medication effects outside of clinical trials: new-user designs. Am J Epidemiol 158(9):915–920
19. Stürmer T, Wyss R, Glynn RJ, Brookhart MA (2014) Propensity scores for confounder adjustment when assessing the effects of medical interventions using nonexperimental study designs. J Intern Med 275(6):570–580

20. Riis AH, Johansen MB, Jacobsen JB et al (2015) Short look-back periods in pharmacoepide-miologic studies of new users of antibiotics and asthma medications introduce severe misclas-sification. Pharmacoepidemiol Drug Saf 24(5):478–485
21. Leslie RS Using arrays to calculate medication utilization. Available at http://www2.sas.com/proceedings/forum2007/043-2007.pdf. Accessed 29 Dec 2015
22. Kleinbaum DG, Kupper LL, Nizam A, Muller KE (2008) Applied regression analysis and other multivariable methods, 4th edn. Duxbury, Belmont
23. Johnson ES, Bartman BA, Briesacher BA et al (2013) The incident user design in comparative effectiveness research. Pharmacoepidemiol Drug Saf 22(1):1–6
24. Harris AD, McGregor JC, Perencevich EN et al (2006) The use and interpretation of quasi-experimental studies in medical informatics. J Am Med Inform Assoc 13(1):16–23
25. Storm A, Andersen SE, Benfeldt E, Serup J (2008) One in 3 prescriptions are never redeemed: primary nonadherence in an outpatient clinic. J Am Acad Dermatol 59(1):27–33
26. Strom BL (2013) Overview of automated databases in pharmacoepidemiology. In: Strom BL, Kimmel SE, Hennessy S (eds) Textbook of pharmacoepidemiology. Wiley-Blackwell, Chichester
27. Lauffenburger JC, Balasubramanian A, Farley JF et al (2013) Completeness of prescription information in US commercial claims databases. Pharmacoepidemiol Drug Saf 22(8):899–906
28. Carstensen SE, Huang KE, Feldman SR (2014) Treatment failure of patients using topical acne treatments: a retrospective observational cohort study. J Dermatolog Treat 25(3):193–195

Chapter 6
Measuring Adherence in Clinical Trials

Scott A. Davis and Steven R. Feldman

Measuring adherence is an essential, but often overlooked, part of clinical trials. As recognition of the importance of adherence for good outcomes has grown, investigators designing clinical trials have tried to maximize adherence, so that patients' poor adherence does not make a drug look less efficacious than it actually is. Luckily, clinical trials have some built-in features that tend to keep adherence relatively high: frequent visits contributing to close monitoring (Hawthorne effect [1]) and the way that clinical trials tend to select for more motivated patients [2]. Nonetheless, adherence in clinical trials remains far from perfect, so measuring patients' use of medication in the trial is helpful to define how well the drug is likely to work in the context of varying adherence patterns [3]. Some drugs have greater "forgiveness" than others, allowing patients to miss occasional doses without significant loss of treatment response [4]. While a drug's forgiveness is likely to be known from pharmacokinetic studies, measuring adherence will still provide vital data on how the drug is likely to work when patients do not use it perfectly [4].

In dermatology, there is often the added difficulty that the way topical medications are used can vary immensely from patient to patient. For example, sun protection factor (SPF) of a sunscreen is calculated based on the assumption of using 2 mg/cm^2 [5]. In everyday practice, patients use less than half this amount [6, 7], neglect to reapply it when needed, and tend to miss certain areas of the skin entirely [8]. A sunscreen with an official SPF of 30 may have a true SPF of only 2 to 3 when used as patients typically use it [9, 10]. Thus, manufacturers are left with a dilemma.

S.A. Davis (✉)
Department of Dermatology, Wake Forest School of Medicine, Winston-Salem, NC, USA

Division of Pharmaceutical Outcomes and Policy, University of North Carolina Eshelman School of Pharmacy, Chapel Hill, NC, USA
e-mail: sdavis81@email.unc.edu

S.R. Feldman
Departments of Dermatology, Pathology, and Public Health Sciences, Wake Forest School of Medicine, Winston-Salem, NC, USA

© Springer International Publishing Switzerland 2016
S.A. Davis (ed.), *Adherence in Dermatology*,
DOI 10.1007/978-3-319-30994-1_6

They can release a dosage that meets the needs of average patients, but may be too high and give too many side effects for fully adherent patients [11]. Alternatively, they can release a lower dosage that is right for fully adherent patients, but too low for the average patient to obtain much efficacy [11]. Variation and ambiguity in the instructions that physicians give (e.g., "use liberally" or "use sparingly") further compound this problem. Not surprisingly, many dermatologists now lean toward reducing the potential for human error by emphasizing sun-protective clothing more often than sunscreen.

6.1 Methods of Adherence Measurement

Ideally, a method for measuring adherence in clinical trials would be objective, accurate, and detailed. Subjective methods are vulnerable to patients' imperfect ability to record or recall doses correctly, as well as their tendency to tell the physician what they believe the physician wants to hear (see Chap. 7 for more details on the psychology of the physician-patient relationship). Subjective methods include patient diaries, direct questioning during visits, and questionnaires such as the Morisky Medication Adherence Scale. Pill counts or medication weights are less subjective in theory, but can still be manipulated by patients who dump out unused pills or creams to give the impression of better adherence [12]. Similarly, electronic diaries and photographic documentation (in which the patient sends a photograph of their medication taking) are possible [11], but these also require full patient cooperation.

Objective methods include biological markers of medication intake (such as levels of drug in the blood), pharmacy refill records, and electronic monitoring. For most drugs, biological markers are less than optimal because the patient may take the drug well just before the blood test visit (white-coat adherence [13]) and have a high concentration of drug at the time of the visit while being poorly adherent at other times. In addition, biological markers are generally useless for topical therapies, which have minimal systemic absorption, and are thus less useful in dermatology. Biological markers are sometimes more useful in trials where a caregiver makes unannounced visits to the patient's home, circumventing the white-coat adherence effect [14].

Pharmacy refills are objective and generally considered a high-quality method of adherence monitoring. Their main drawback is that they do not give detailed data on the timing of dose omissions. In addition, pharmacy refills do not guarantee that the medication was actually taken. Some patients stockpile doses, or even give or sell medications illegally to others, causing pharmacy refills to give a false impression of perfect adherence.

A method that has the benefits of being both objective and detailed is electronic monitoring. Most commonly, electronic monitoring consists of a cap with a computer chip inside, such as the Medication Event Monitoring System (MEMS®) cap

September 2007								October 2007						
Mon	Tue	Wed	Thr	Fri	Sat	Sun		Mon	Tue	Wed	Thr	Fri	Sat	Sun
								1 2	2 2	3 1				
		5 3	6 3	7 2	8 2	9 2								
10 2	11 3	12 2	13 2	14 2	15 2	16 2								
17 2	18 3	19 3	20 2	21 2	22 2	23 2								
24 2	25 2	26 2	27 2	28 2	29 2	30 2								

Fig. 6.1 Calendar report showing a patient's adherence as number of doses taken on each date

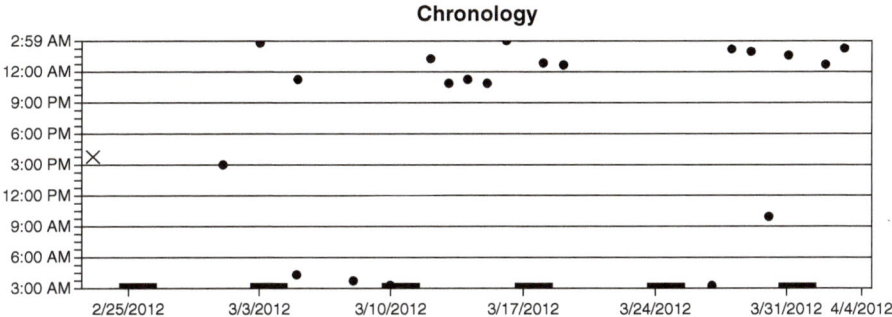

Fig. 6.2 Timing report highlighting a patient's routine as measured by the time of day each dose was taken. *X* indicates event excluded from calculations (i.e., when the medication was dispensed or collected)

(MWV Healthcare, Sion, Switzerland). This can be used with an adapter for topical medication tubes [15] and can even be used to monitor adherence to injectable treatments, such as biologics, by placing the cap on a large empty bottle labeled as a disposal container for used syringes [16].

Electronic monitors use a sensor to record the day and time that the container of medication is opened or closed. The cap can then be collected at visits and read through a reader connected to a computer. Software then generates reports on each patient's adherence, such as a calendar report (Fig. 6.1) showing the number of doses taken on each day or a timing report (Fig. 6.2) showing a marker for each time the medication was taken. The timing report is most useful to draw attention to whether the patient has a routine of taking the medication at the same time(s) every day. The software can also automatically calculate measures such as percent of expected doses taken and percent of days with correct dosing.

Electronic monitoring also exists in other forms, such as "smart pills," which actually contain a device within the pill that responds to stomach juices, sending a signal to the person monitoring the medication intake [11]. Smart pill boxes or blister packs automatically recording the time of opening are also available. As of the time of this writing, no literature was found indicating that any of these methods have been used in dermatology trials. However, one trial did use a data logger on a phototherapy device to measure adherence to home phototherapy for psoriasis [17].

Trials using both electronic monitoring and patient diaries have confirmed that about 26 % of patient-reported doses are not verified by the electronic monitors [18, 19]. Electronic monitoring has been used in dermatology to show that adherence rises around the time of office visits [20] and to compare interventions for improving adherence to acne treatments [21–23] and sunscreen [24].

6.2   Stealth Electronic Monitoring

One problem with monitoring adherence in clinical trials is that when patients know they are being monitored, it may change their behavior, a form of Hawthorne effect [1]. For trials of new drugs, this may be beneficial, as the goal is to find out how effective the drug is when it is used; maximizing adherence by any means, including via Hawthorne effects, should be helpful in this regard. In trials designed to better understand what adherence behavior is like in normal patient populations, the Hawthorne effect is a weakness. When it is necessary to mimic real-world conditions most closely, avoiding Hawthorne effects on behavior, stealth monitoring can be used.

Stealth monitoring, in which patients are not told until the end of the trial that they are being monitored, is likely to be the most accurate measure of how patients normally behave. [2] Although stealth monitoring could be considered unethical under certain circumstances, the stealth monitoring may be the only way to get accurate data on patients' real-world behavior and can be ethical when the benefits outweigh the risks (Table 6.1) [2]. Under US human subjects' protection regulations, deceptive approaches are permitted if their benefits outweigh their risks, and alternative nondeceptive approaches are not feasible. Even in studies in which patients will only receive standard-of-care medical treatments, stealth monitoring has risks. These risks may be outweighed when benefits of knowing patients' actual real-world adherence behavior are important. These benefits may accrue both to the individual patient being treated and to society at large. Knowing whether patients are adherent to a standard, low-risk medication, such as topical adapalene for acne or topical clobetasol for psoriasis, also has the benefit that it can help keep patients off more dangerous systemic medications, such as isotretinoin or systemic psoriasis treatments [2]. If adherence is low, then counseling patients about better adherence can improve their outcomes without escalating them to a more dangerous medication.

Table 6.1 Possible pitfalls to stealth electronic monitoring trials and possible solutions

Potential pitfall	Solution
Not informing patients about the electronic monitoring carries a risk of psychological impact to some patients and a risk that public confidence in researchers could be reduced	State that the benefit of knowing whether treatment failure was caused by poor adherence outweighs the risk of psychological effects on subjects. Most patients are not bothered by having their adherence electronically monitored, provided the results are used for their benefit
	If we find that poor adherence is causing treatment failure, we can avoid escalation to a more dangerous treatment
	Share the results of patients as a group, so that patients do not feel singled out if they have had poor adherence
Patients need to be informed that they are being monitored	Inform subjects that they are being monitored and that their medication will be weighed or pills will be counted at visits. However, the presence of the electronic monitor is not disclosed until the end of the trial
Stealth monitoring is a deceptive approach	Other nondeceptive approaches are not feasible because they would not provide accurate data on patients' real-world behaviors. The deception will be disclosed at the end of the trial
	When the deception is disclosed at end of study, consent from patients can be obtained to look at the adherence data. That way, patients give consent before the data are seen, but the data are not biased by the monitoring procedure. However, this approach runs the risk of bias, as highly nonadherent patients could be more likely to refuse to provide consent. If it were sufficiently critical to obtain adherence data on all participants, monitoring could be done without giving study subjects the opportunity to limit access to the data

6.3 When Electronic Monitoring Is Not Feasible

Occasionally electronic monitoring in a clinical trial is not feasible. If medication is being dispensed from sources not under the investigators' control, it may not be possible to attach an electronic monitor to the medication, or if subjects are not scheduled for regular return visits, it may not be possible to collect electronic monitors. In these cases, pharmacy refill records may be the best source of adherence data. If pharmacy refills cannot be used either, measuring disease outcomes at a follow-up visit may be helpful, although they give only an indirect measure of adherence.

6.4 Limitations of Electronic Monitoring

Although electronic monitoring is currently considered the gold standard for adherence monitoring, electronic monitoring does have a few limitations. Electronic monitoring cannot guarantee that a medication removed from the container was necessarily consumed. If patients prefer to use a pill box, then the medication container may be opened less frequently and multiple doses may be removed at one time. Patients may forget to replace the cap when they use a dose, and some may not return the cap to have it read. Using electronic monitoring together with another method, such as pharmacy refills, pill counts, or direct questioning about the way the patient uses the medication, might help address some of these limitations. For example, a patient who opens the container once a week, at precisely the same time every week, may be using a pill box. If this patient has perfect adherence according to pharmacy refills or pill counts, they probably have excellent adherence facilitated by the pill box.

6.5 Conclusion

Despite these limitations, electronic monitoring is the best method currently available for gathering accurate adherence data in clinical trials. Measuring adherence in a trial can provide more detailed information on how a medication works in real-world settings, where perfect adherence cannot be expected.

References

1. Davis SA, Feldman SR (2013) Using Hawthorne effects to improve adherence in clinical practice: lessons from clinical trials. JAMA Dermatol 149(4):490–491
2. Krejci-Manwaring J, Tusa M, Carroll CL et al (2007) Stealth monitoring of adherence to topical medication: adherence is very poor in children with atopic dermatitis. J Am Acad Dermatol 56:211–216
3. Vrijens B, Vincze G, Kristanto P, Urquhart J, Burnier M (2008) Adherence to prescribed antihypertensive drug treatments: longitudinal study of electronically compiled dosing histories. BMJ 336(7653):1114–1117
4. Urquhart J (1998) Pharmacodynamics of variable patient compliance: implications for pharmaceutical value. Adv Drug Deliv Rev 33(3):207–219
5. US Food and Drug Administration (2012) Labeling and effectiveness testing: sunscreen drug products for over-the-counter human use – small entity compliance guide. http://www.fda.gov/drugs/guidancecomplianceregulatoryinformation/guidances/ucm330694.htm. Accessed 13 May 2014
6. Autier P, Boniol M, Severi G, Dore JF (2001) Quantity of sunscreen used by European students. Br J Dermatol 144(2):288–291
7. Neale R, Williams G, Green A (2002) Application patterns among participants randomized to daily sunscreen use in a skin cancer prevention trial. Arch Dermatol 138(10):1319–1325
8. Ulff E, Maroti M, Kettis-Lindblad A et al (2007) Single application of a fluorescent test cream by healthy volunteers: assessment of treated and neglected body sites. Br J Dermatol 156(5):974–978
9. Schalka S, dos Reis VM, Cuce LC (2009) The influence of the amount of sunscreen applied and its sun protection factor (SPF): evaluation of two sunscreens including the same ingredients at different concentrations. Photodermatol Photoimmunol Photomed 25(4):175–180

10. Kim SM, Oh BH, Lee YW, Choe YB, Ahn KJ (2010) The relation between the amount of sunscreen applied and the sun protection factor in Asian skin. J Am Acad Dermatol 62(2):218–222
11. Vrijens B, Urquhart J (2014) Methods for measuring, enhancing, and accounting for medication adherence in clinical trials. Clin Pharmacol Ther 10 95(6):617–626
12. Feldman SR (2009) Practical ways to improve patients' treatment outcomes. Medical Quality Enhancement Corporation, Winston-Salem
13. Feinstein AR (1990) On white-coat effects and the electronic monitoring of compliance. Arch Intern Med 150(7):1377–1378
14. Capgemini Consulting (2011) Patient adherence: the next frontier in patient care. http://adhereforhealth.org/wpcontent/uploads/pdf/Patient_Adherence__The_Next_Frontier_in_Patient_Care%20-%20CapGemini_2011.pdf. (Accessed 3 Mar 2016)
15. Tusa MG, Ladd M, Kaur M, Balkrishnan R, Feldman SR (2006) Adapting electronic adherence monitors to standard packages of topical medications. J Am Acad Dermatol 55(5):886–887
16. West C, Narahari S, O'Neill J et al (2013) Adherence to adalimumab in patients with moderate to severe psoriasis. Dermatol Online J 19(5):18182
17. Yentzer BA, Yelverton CB, Pearce DJ et al (2008) Adherence to acitretin and home narrow-band ultraviolet B phototherapy in patients with psoriasis. J Am Acad Dermatol 59(4):577–581
18. Balkrishnan R, Carroll CL, Camacho FT, Feldman SR (2003) Electronic monitoring of medication adherence in skin disease: results of a pilot study. J Am Acad Dermatol 49(4):651–654
19. Carroll CL, Feldman SR, Camacho FT, Manuel JM, Balkrishnan R (2004) Adherence to topical therapy decreases over the course of an 8-week psoriasis clinical trial: commonly used methods of measuring adherence to topical therapy overestimate actual use. J Am Acad Dermatol 51(2):212–216
20. Feldman SR, Camacho FT, Krejci-Manwaring J, Carroll CL, Balkrishnan R (2007) Adherence to topical therapy increases around the time of office visits. J Am Acad Dermatol 57(1):81–83
21. Yentzer BA, Gosnell AL, Clark AR et al (2011) A randomized controlled pilot study of strategies to increase adherence in teenagers with acne vulgaris. J Am Acad Dermatol 64(4):793–795
22. Yentzer BA, Wood AA, Sagransky MJ et al (2011) An internet-based survey and improvement of acne treatment outcomes. Arch Dermatol 147(10):1223–1224
23. Boker A, Feetham HJ, Armstrong A, Purcell P, Jacobe H (2012) Do automated text messages increase adherence to acne therapy? Results of a randomized, controlled trial. J Am Acad Dermatol 67(6):1136–1142
24. Armstrong AW, Watson AJ, Makredes M, Frangos JE, Kimball AB, Kvedar JC (2009) Text-message reminders to improve sunscreen use: a randomized, controlled trial using electronic monitoring. Arch Dermatol 145(11):1230–1236

Chapter 7
How Providers Can Assess Their Patients' Adherence in Clinical Settings

Scott A. Davis and Steven R. Feldman

While large databases are excellent tools for studying patterns of adherence in large populations, and electronic monitoring gives valuable data in clinical trials, different methods are needed to ascertain patients' adherence behavior in the clinical setting. Electronic monitors are too expensive (generally US$100–150) for everyday clinical use, and many patients would not consent to be electronically monitored. Therefore, clinicians need to be conscious of how to question patients to get useful data on adherence patterns [1].

There are direct self-report tools, such as the Morisky Medication Adherence Scale, that can be used to query patients about adherence. These are of very limited value. For example, the version of the Morisky scale most commonly used today consists of eight questions, asking patients about which days they take medication, how often they forget to take it or bring it with them when traveling, and whether they have cut back without telling their doctor (Table 7.1) [2]. Some studies have shown correlations of R^2 less than 0.2 between results from the Morisky scale and medication refill adherence, one of the most reliable measures [3]. While an R^2 of 0.2 might be rather impressive for a variable that is only one of many independent variables influencing a dependent variable, it is extremely low when correlating two measures that purport to measure the same thing. For a scale to serve as an adequate proxy for an unmeasured quantity, the R^2 needs to be very close to 1. Thus, we do not consider this type of self-report scale to have adequate reliability for informing decision-making.

S.A. Davis (✉)
Department of Dermatology, Wake Forest School of Medicine, Winston-Salem, NC, USA

Division of Pharmaceutical Outcomes and Policy, University of North Carolina Eshelman School of Pharmacy, Chapel Hill, NC, USA
e-mail: sdavis81@email.unc.edu

S.R. Feldman
Departments of Dermatology, Pathology, and Public Health Sciences, Wake Forest School of Medicine, Winston-Salem, NC, USA

© Springer International Publishing Switzerland 2016
S.A. Davis (ed.), *Adherence in Dermatology*,
DOI 10.1007/978-3-319-30994-1_7

7.1 Why Direct Self-Report Is Not Reliable: Insights from Social Psychology

Social psychology suggests that people will often avoid conflict by giving the answer they expect the listener will want to hear [4, 5]. In many cases, they do not believe the listener wants to hear the whole truth, but instead would prefer to hear a socially acceptable answer (social desirability bias) [6]. Since clinicians actually need accurate information to make sound decisions, it is important to know how to induce accurate disclosure of patients' nonadherence to improve decision-making (Table 7.2) [7].

Accurate clinical assessment of nonadherence includes understanding of the patient's motive for using or not using the medication, which is also not reliably collected by self-report. Since reminder approaches are useful for forgetfulness, but not very useful for intentional nonadherence, it is important not to misclassify intentional nonadherence as unintentional. Actually, when asked about their reasons for nonadherence in an anonymous survey, only 24 % cite forgetting as their reason for not using the drug [8].

The idea that only a minority of patients are nonadherent due to forgetfulness may seem at odds with what clinicians are accustomed to hearing from patients. Saying that they forgot is much less stressful to patients than challenging authority

Table 7.1 Eight-item Morisky Medication Adherence Scale (as originally validated for hypertension) [2]

1. Do you sometimes forget to take your high blood pressure pills?
2. Over the past 2 weeks, were there any days when you did not take your high blood pressure medications?
3. Have you ever cut back or stopped taking your medication without telling your doctor because you felt worse when you took it?
4. When you travel or leave home, do you sometimes forget to bring along your medications?
5. Did you take your high blood pressure medicine yesterday?
6. When you feel like your blood pressure is under control, do you sometimes stop taking your medicine?
7. Taking medication everyday [sic] is a real inconvenience for some people. Do you ever feel hassled about sticking to your blood pressure treatment plan?
8. How often do you have difficulty remembering to take all your blood pressure medication?

Table 7.2 Problems with relying on direct self-report of medication use

Patients' poor memory or recall of past events
Patients deceive themselves into thinking they are good adherers and then communicate their genuine but false belief to the clinician
Patient wants to avoid conflict by not disclosing their low adherence
Patient wants to avoid conflict by suggesting a more socially acceptable reason (e.g., forgetting) rather than not wanting to use the medication
Patient misunderstands the regimen and thinks they are executing it well when they are not

by stating a reason that may create a feeling of conflict with the clinician [4, 9]. People's tendency to submit to authority is often underestimated, but is well documented in psychology from the Milgram experiments – showing that subjects would obey the experimenter even to the point of administering a near-fatal electric shock – all the way up to the present day [10]. People are also socialized not to share the whole truth to sustain harmonious social relationships, especially with those of higher status. Instead, people are taught to tell "little white lies" such as, "Your house is lovely!" or "You are such a great cook!" [11]. Indeed, results from anonymous surveys and objective electronic monitors hidden in the caps of medication bottles reveal that patients greatly overreport their adherence and give socially acceptable but misleading reasons when asked to explain their nonadherence in clinical settings [12]. Not only do patients want to look good to physicians, they also want to look good to themselves. Sometimes patients lie to themselves and then tell the physician their genuine (but false) belief that they are adherent [13].

In a physician-patient relationship, the patient is normally acutely aware of the profound inequality in medical and pharmacological knowledge, power, and status. This inequality unsurprisingly contributes to incomplete disclosure of the patient's perspective [7]. At the same time, patients generally have strong commitments to certain preferences and worldviews, which are not easily changed and prevent patients from easily yielding to the view of someone with more knowledge (Table 7.3). At least in countries with a tradition of valuing equality, they want to be treated as equals, even when they know that the physician is much more knowledgeable. Moreover, patients become even more committed to defend their preexisting worldviews when they feel that they are being coerced to do something different [14–16].

In medical education, increasingly curricula are being reworked to ensure that the physician knows how to extract patient's perspectives that will not be disclosed until the patient feels it is safe [7]. Medical students now learn that patients are, in a sense, the experts on their own illnesses [9] and that a physician must do everything possible to ensure that potential motives for future intentional nonadherence do not remain secret. Motivational interviewing (see Chap. 16) attempts to minimize feelings of conflict by eliciting the patient's self-generated ideas about potential

Table 7.3 Different patient worldviews that influence patient behavior

Trait	Agreeable type of patient	Skeptical type
View of medications	Likes medication because a medication makes them feel safe	Dislikes medication because a medication reminds them they have a problem [17]
View of physician visits	Likes seeing a physician frequently, even when healthy	Avoids seeing a physician for as long as possible
View of symptoms	Is very concerned about the slightest abnormality	Is proud that they can withstand substantial pain without complaint
Willingness to admit own weaknesses	Is willing to admit limitations such as inability to afford a medication or not knowing how to use the medication	Wants to "save face" with the physician rather than disclosing limitations

treatment and then responding accordingly [18]. If the patient is truly not motivated
to treat the illness at all, motivational interviewing may reveal quickly that trying to
push a treatment on the patient is futile [7]. Models of behavior change define several
stages, beginning with the precontemplative stage, in which a person is not yet
prepared to take any action. If the patient is past the precontemplative stage, their
actual motivational drives can be investigated and used to negotiate a mutually
agreeable solution.

7.2   Promoting Frank and Open Disclosure

Normalizing the patient's likely behavior is perhaps the most fundamental strategy
to make patients comfortable with stating their true patterns of taking medication.
Try saying something like, "Most patients have trouble remembering to take their
medications every day. How often do you usually miss a dose?" This way, patients
may be proud to say that they miss only two days a week [6, 9, 19]. Kjellgren and
colleagues suggest adding, "When do you feel a need to change the way you use
your medications?" [6] Some may feel this approach goes too far in the direction of
condoning changes in the regimen without physician consultation, but for some
regimens, it may be helpful.

If dealing with adolescents, try to assess their perspective without their parents
in the room [9]. In one pilot study, calling adolescents' parents to remind them to
use an acne medication led to lower adherence than a control group that was not
reminded at all [20]. These results reveal how adolescents are determined to assert
their independence against parents who insist on treatment, even if it means suffering
with more acne [19].

Although telling the whole truth about their low adherence is often stressful to
patients, keeping up appearances is stressful as well, underscoring the importance
of normalizing the patient's likely behavior so they can disclose it honestly. One of
the authors (Feldman) has written of his experience with scalp psoriasis patients:

> I had been invited to give a lecture at a National Psoriasis Foundation national meeting for
> patients on the topic of scalp psoriasis treatment. The venue was a large room filled with
> rows and rows of patients with scalp psoriasis. Standing at the podium, I began: "Scalp
> psoriasis is so frustrating." This opening was meant to let the patients in the room know they
> were listening to a caring, empathetic doctor. The entire room of heads nodded in agreement.
> "It is not just frustrating for patients; it's frustrating for us dermatologists, too. We
> like to see our patients get well, and scalp psoriasis just never seems to get better." Again,
> the room of heads nodded in agreement. "I think I know why it's not getting better," I said.
> The entire audience was quiet, heads peered forward, eyes wide open, seeking to learn why
> scalp psoriasis doesn't go away. I raised my hand, pointed at the group and said: "Because
> you're not putting the medication on your heads."
>
>   Throughout the entire room, heads fell to chests with a great collective sigh of catharsis.
> "Yes," these patients thought, "I haven't been using the medication, and it feels so good to
> get it off my chest. I have been lying to my doctor about this for so long. It feels good to
> finally admit this to a doctor." [19]

Table 7.4 Behavioral economics strategies to reduce dishonesty

Strategy	Examples
Reminder of ethical principles	Study subjects asked to recall the Ten Commandments were more honest when reporting their results in a matrix-completion task. In clinical settings, patients could be asked about their religious affiliation before asking adherence questions
Signing a pledge to report honestly	On a car insurance application, people who signed a pledge of accuracy at the top of the page reported more accurate mileage driven, compared to those who signed the same pledge when it was placed at the bottom of the page
Establish honesty as an ingroup norm and appeal to group membership	Students cheated less if they observed an outgroup member (a student from a rival university) cheating during the experiment

7.3   Improving Honesty: Insights from Behavioral Economics

Behavioral economists have investigated ways to improve honesty. On a matrix-completion task used in psychological studies, participants normally tend to cheat by exaggerating their results by about 15 % [11]. Dan Ariely hypothesized that a rational choice theory of cheating – in which the level of cheating depends solely on the likelihood and consequences of being caught – could not explain the level of dishonesty [11]. Instead, the person's internal moral compass was more important, though it allowed a disturbing amount of rationalization. People could cheat up to about 15 % and still rationalize that there was nothing wrong with their behavior, but beyond that, they would start to feel they were doing wrong.

Dishonesty is significantly reduced when a context of honesty is invoked (Table 7.4). In Ariely's studies, asking participants to recall some of the Ten Commandments completely eliminated dishonest behavior, regardless of the participant's religion [11]. Thinking about the Ten Commandments made the idea of honesty salient, preventing people from being able to lie and still think of themselves as good people.

7.4   Indirect Strategies to Assess Adherence

Thus far we have described ways to make the patient feel safe in disclosing their actual adherence behavior honestly or improve honesty with the proper context. Some patients will still tend not to disclose their low adherence, especially if they never obtained the medication or quit taking it very early. For these patients, often indirect questioning techniques, or strategies that cause the patient to inadvertently admit low adherence, are helpful. At the simplest level, these strategies can involve asking patients about the name or color of their medication, which they may not know if they never filled the prescription or have not used it in a long time [21, 22].

Other questions may hint at when the last refill took place, what the patient is doing with accumulated medication, or how the patient disposes of medication (see Table in Ref. [23]) [19, 23]. Patients who are adherent should have a refill within the expected time frame and should not be accumulating or having to dispose of medication. This strategy can also sometimes reveal cases in which the patient thought they were using the medication correctly, but actually misunderstood the prescribed regimen [24]. Asking the patient exactly what they were supposed to do is especially effective in determining whether we communicated the instructions well at the prior visit.

If we ask patients to bring their medication to the visit, we can look to see if the tube or bottle is still full [19]. If it is completely empty, chances are that the patient dumped it in the toilet. If we prescribe a few more pills than we expect the patient to use, such as 70 pills for QD use and see the patient back in 60 days, then we know there should be 10 pills remaining [19]. If there are none remaining, the patient probably dumped it out.

Patients who say things like, "You're seeing my acne on a good day; usually it is worse than this," may be revealing a pattern of "white-coat adherence," [25] where they took the medication only on the few days before the visit. This phenomenon is similar to dental floss or piano lessons, where people floss or practice piano only on the few days before seeing the dentist or piano teacher. Scheduling an early return visit at 3 days or 1 week can help get these patients into a regular habit of taking the medication. The aim is to cause patients to take the medication very well for the first week, persuading them that the medication is highly effective and worth taking, even when the physician is not monitoring them so closely.

Some patients may also give us clues by casually admitting that they have non-dermatologic chronic conditions such as hypertension or high cholesterol, but are not taking medication for the comorbid condition. Past behavior is the best predictor of future behavior, and a patient who does not adhere to one medication is likely to behave the same way with other medications [1, 26]. This type of patient would probably not admit to their primary care provider that they are nonadherent to their antihypertensive or cholesterol medications, but may feel very comfortable admitting the same fact to their dermatologist. By asking about their medical history, we may be able to reveal whether the patient is a health-conscious type of person. If not, we would probably do well to assume that they are not very adherent.

Sometimes we just need to read between the lines and derive the right message from a cryptic statement the patient made. For example, "It didn't work" generally means that either the patient never tried it or they used it for a while and then stopped and saw the disease come back [9]. We could follow up with a question like, "Did it work for a while, and then it stopped working?" If the patient says yes, then it is likely that they saw some improvement and then stopped using the medication, allowing the disease to come back. We should be sure to educate these patients on the way that many treatments for skin diseases are not "cures," and therefore continued use of maintenance therapy is crucial.

References

1. DiMatteo MR, Haskard-Zolnierek KB, Martin LR (2012) Improving patient adherence: a three-factor model to guide practice. Health Psychol Rev 6(1):74–91
2. Morisky DE, Ang A, Krousel-Wood M, Ward HJ (2008) Predictive validity of a medication adherence measure in an outpatient setting. J Clin Hypertens (Greenwich) 10(5):348–354
3. Wang Y, Kong MC, Ko Y (2013) Comparison of three medication adherence measures in patients taking warfarin. J Thromb Thrombolysis 36(4):416–421
4. Palmieri JJ, Stern TA (2009) Lies in the doctor-patient relationship. Prim Care Companion J Clin Psychiatry 11(4):163–168
5. Grover SL (1993) Lying, deceit, and subterfuge: a model of dishonesty in the workplace. Organ Sci 4(3):478–495
6. Kjellgren KI, Ring L, Lindblad AK, Maroti M, Serup J (2004) To follow dermatological treatment regimens – patients' and providers' views. Acta Derm Venereol 84(6):445–450
7. Cole SA, Bird J (2000) The medical interview: the three-function approach, 2nd edn. Mosby, St. Louis
8. Frost & Sullivan (2005) Patient nonadherence: tools for combating persistence and compliance issues. http://www.frost.com/prod/servlet/cpo/115071625.pdf. Accessed 6 May 2014
9. Baldwin HE (2006) Tricks for improving compliance with acne therapy. Dermatol Ther 19(4):224–236
10. Milgram S (1963) Behavioral study of obedience. J Abnorm Soc Psychol 67(4):371–378
11. Ariely D (2012) The (honest) truth about dishonesty: how we lie to everyone – especially ourselves. HarperCollins, New York
12. Balkrishnan R, Carroll CL, Camacho FT, Feldman SR (2003) Electronic monitoring of medication adherence in skin disease: results of a pilot study. J Am Acad Dermatol 49(4):651–654
13. Reddy S (2013) 'I Don't Smoke, Doc,' and other patient lies. http://online.wsj.com/news/articles/SB10001424127887323478004578306510461212692?mod=health_newsreel&mg=reno64-wsj&url=http%3A%2F%2Fonline.wsj.com%2Farticle%2FSB10001424127887323478004578306510461212692html%3Fmod%3Dhealth_newsreel. Accessed 21 May 2014
14. Aslam I, Davis SA, Feldman SR (2014) Resisting ideas of others. In: Davis SA, Feldman SR (eds) An illustrated dictionary of behavioral economics for healthcare professionals. CreateSpace, Charleston
15. Lehane E, McCarthy G (2007) Intentional and unintentional medication non-adherence: a comprehensive framework for clinical research and practice? A discussion paper. Int J Nurs Stud 44(8):1468–1477
16. Fogarty JS (1997) Reactance theory and patient noncompliance. Soc Sci Med 45(8):1277–1288
17. Hugtenburg JG, Timmers L, Elders PJ, Vervloet M, van Dijk L (2013) Definitions, variants, and causes of nonadherence with medication: a challenge for tailored interventions. Patient Prefer Adherence 7:675–682. doi:10.2147/PPA.S29549.Print;%2013.:675–682
18. Rollnick S, Butler CC, Kinnersley P, Gregory J, Mash B (2010) Motivational interviewing. BMJ 340:c1900. doi:10.1136/bmj.c1900.:c1900
19. Feldman SR (2009) Practical ways to improve patients' treatment outcomes. Medical Quality Enhancement Corporation, Winston-Salem
20. Yentzer BA, Gosnell AL, Clark AR et al (2011) A randomized controlled pilot study of strategies to increase adherence in teenagers with acne vulgaris. J Am Acad Dermatol 64(4):793–795
21. Jones-Caballero M, Pedrosa E, Penas PF (2008) Self-reported adherence to treatment and quality of life in mild to moderate acne. Dermatology 217(4):309–314
22. Pawin H, Beylot C, Chivot M et al (2009) Creation of a tool to assess adherence to treatments for acne. Dermatology 218(1):26–32

23. Alinia H, Feldman SR (2014) Assessing medication adherence using indirect self-report. JAMA Dermatol 150(8):813–814
24. Stephenson BJ, Rowe BH, Haynes RB, Macharia WM, Leon G (1993) The rational clinical examination. Is this patient taking the treatment as prescribed? JAMA 269(21):2779–2781
25. Feinstein AR (1990) On white-coat effects and the electronic monitoring of compliance. Arch Intern Med 150(7):1377–1378
26. Sherbourne CD, Hays RD, Ordway L, DiMatteo MR, Kravitz RL (1992) Antecedents of adherence to medical recommendations: results from the Medical Outcomes Study. J Behav Med 15(5):447–468

Chapter 8
Topical Application and Variability of the De Facto Applied Dose: Technical Aspects

Dina Vind-Kezunovic and Jørgen Vedelskov Serup

8.1 Introduction

Topical treatment of skin disease is rational because the active substance is applied directly to the target skin area thus with minimal systemic exposure. However, accurate dosing of a given formulation (cream, ointment, solution, or gel) can be difficult to control for individuals with cognitive or psychological dysfunction and physical deficits such as impaired vision or joint problems. Also factors such as forgetfulness, neglect, and a stressful life can interfere with applications.

In this chapter, we focus on the technical aspects of self-application of motivated individuals being in a good mental, psychological, and physical condition, who received detailed information on how to apply. Already back in 1964, it was shown by Schlagel and Sanborn in the *Journal of Investigative Dermatology* that repeated instruction plays a major role [1]. The well-instructed operator not only performs a better application technique compared to a superficially informed person but can also apply reproducible weights of ointments or creams to the body. Variation of application both has intrapersonal and interpersonal aspects. The recommended standard dose expressed by the drug company, the doctor, or derived from a guideline is sensitive to both aspects.

But what is the best treatment scenario? Do well-instructed motivated healthy volunteers apply the recommended amounts of topical medication the same? Is there a topical formulation of choice with less variation? Does the applied local

D. Vind-Kezunovic
Department of Dermatology, St. Olav's University Hospital, Trondheim, Norway
e-mail: dinavind@hotmail.com

J.V. Serup (✉)
Department of Dermatology, Bispebjerg University Hospital,
Copenhagen, Denmark
e-mail: Joergen.vedelskov.serup@regionh.dk

© Springer International Publishing Switzerland 2016
S.A. Davis (ed.), *Adherence in Dermatology*,
DOI 10.1007/978-3-319-30994-1_8

dose depend on the treated anatomical site? Are some anatomical sites prone to be completely neglected?

8.2   Even Spreadability Depends on the Topical Formulation

The fingertip unit has been suggested to be a practical dosage standard for ointment as described by Long and Finlay in 1991 [2]. However, the validation of this unit has been lacking for the less viscous vehicles including cream, gel, and solution. A fingertip unit (FTU) is the amount of ointment expressed from a tube with a 5-mm diameter nozzle, applied from the distal skin crease to the tip of the index finger [2]. A recent study aimed to investigate how evenly healthy individuals were able to apply four different pharmaceutical vehicles to the abdomen [3]. The participants were instructed to spread the formulation from a defined spot centrifugally on the abdomen the way they would normally apply a skin product. They were to apply 0.1 g of product corresponding to 0.2 FTU of a test ointment, two different creams (a low-viscosity and a high-viscosity cream, respectively), and an alcoholic solution. The spreadability of the four pharmaceutical vehicles was compared: ointment (actually the vehicle of calcipotriol Daivonex®/Dovonex® with 76.4 % lipid), an ordinary emulsifying cream (with 28.2 % lipid), a low-viscosity cream (with 10 % lipid), and a solution (no lipid but 51 % water and 43 % alcohol). The mean area was measured under ultraviolet light (cm^2) and the applied dose (mg/cm^2) was calculated.

Evenness of application in the field was assessed. Only the ointment was evenly spread leaving a glistening homogenous layer on the skin. This was in contrast to the other vehicles all spread sparsely at the periphery. No difference in the left- or right-side application on the abdomen when using the index finger of the dominant arm was found. Thus, ointment performed best with respect to producing a uniform application film and thus even dosing of the topical.

8.3   Application Technique Depends on the Anatomical Site

Some body sites are obviously more difficult to reach. Consequently a good application technique is less likely to be achieved even for a healthy person in certain sites such as the back. A study investigated the self-application technique and local dose of a test cream applied to 80 % of the total body area (the hairy scalp, head, neck and the body covered by underwear was avoided and not investigated, because local application to these body sites a priori would skew the results) [4]. Healthy Swedish hospital personnel were instructed to apply a fluorescent test cream to the defined large target body area (Fig. 8.1). This test cream had originally been produced as an educational tool for persons with contact dermatitis to help training in application of protective hand creams. It did not emit fluorescence under room conditions but under ultraviolet radiation. The emittance could be read as blue and

Fig. 8.1 Self-application of a fluorescent test cream demonstrated uneven spread of the formulation and neglect of sites on the back of the hand, the armpits, and the skin adjacent to textile

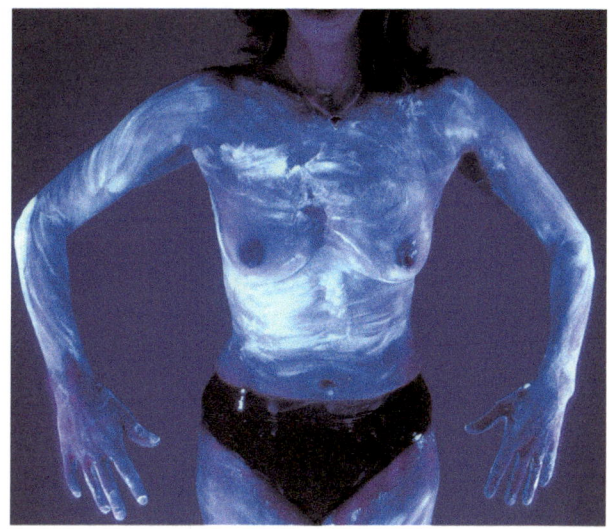

white fluorescence. The trial subjects were told to apply the test cream as they usually would use a cosmetic cream or topical drug. Only a single first application was investigated in the study. A chair was available so that the volunteers could sit down and take their time without being rushed. Subsequently, the target skin area was systematically investigated with a whole body 360° check under ultraviolet illumination. Treated and untreated areas were measured. Overall, 31 % of the target skin surface did not show any fluorescence at all and hence was assumed to have been completely neglected. Typical untreated body sites not surprisingly included the central back (55 %), feet, sole (55 %), upper breast (47 %), leg (29 %), arm (18 %), and hands (15 %). The posterior aspects of both the trunk and the extremities, not easily treated, more often were neglected. In the treated body sites, fluorescence was unevenly distributed and sparse especially close to the textiles, i.e., the underwear. All volunteers were right-handed; no side difference was found. There were no age-related differences. Thus horizontal spread of a topical to large skin fields varies a lot, and some one-third of the skin is completely neglected even if users are completely healthy and motivated. "Difficult zones" can be nominated (see above).

8.4 Well-Instructed Individuals Apply Highly Variable Amounts of Topical Treatment Despite Optimal Conditions and Efforts to Minimize Variation

If all or nearly all major determinants of inaccurate application and poor adherence are taken into account in the study design, is it then possible for users to perform to perfection with little variation in the locally applied dose due to such optimized application strategy? A recent good clinical practice (GCP) study focusing on instruction and monitoring of application reported major variation of the topical dose practiced as twice daily applications over a 3-week study period [5]. The study was blinded and part of a larger clinical trial that aimed to investigate the local tolerability of a 1 % captopril ointment versus a placebo ointment. Trial subjects were asked to use both arms with delineated target test fields of 51 cm^2 on each cubital fossa and antecubital skin. One side was used for the captopril ointment and the other for placebo; hence each person acted as his own control. The placebo test ointment was a pH-neutral, nonaqueous paraffin ointment. Every participant was verified to have a normal physical examination before block randomization. All participants were physically and mentally in a good state, and they were motivated and also paid for their time and active participation.

At the baseline visit, the principal investigator provided the volunteers with oral and written detailed instructions on how to apply the test ointment in a glistening homogenous layer of 2 mg/cm^2. International consensus on sunscreen application often relies on this layer thickness to be the recommended dose [6]. The technical aspects of application were trained under the supervision of the principal investigator at the baseline visit. The weekly objective measurement of adherence was based on weighing the ointment tubes and the data from self-reported diaries. The test areas were marked with green and red pens on the right and left sides, respectively, at the weekly visits. The required adherence for this study was set at 80 % of all evaluated data, including diary entries, results of weighing the tubes, and on the principal investigator's overall evaluation.

There was, nevertheless, a major variation of ointment application ranging from less than 1.96 mg/cm^2 (~100 mg) per application to almost 17.65 mg/cm^2 (~900 mg) per application. A 13.6-fold difference was calculated between the lowest (1.26 mg/cm^2 or ~64.3 mg) and highest application (17.19 mg/cm^2 or ~876.9 mg). The median amount applied was 5.60 mg/cm^2 (~285.7 mg), corresponding to a 2.8-fold increase over the suggested standard application of 2 mg/cm^2. Thus both dosage level and variation were high and very different from what was anticipated in the protocol. Results obtained at weeks 2 and 3 showed the same tendency. The application nadir and zenith at week 2 was 1.66 and 17.93 mg/cm^2, and at week 3 it was 1.26 and 13.89 mg/cm^2. The median was more than double of the standard application value (5.46 mg/cm^2 at visit 2 and 5.08 mg/cm^2 at visit 3). Interestingly, these results are in contrast and even in conflict with another Danish study of dermatology outpatients who were monitored while using topical treatments prescribed in clinical routine and applied by patients in their homes under real conditions. The patients in their homes used as little as median 35 % of the recommended dosage, and 95 % of patients underdosed the treatment [7]. Thus, in the GCP-monitored study, participants applied variably and too much of the test material contrasting the situation of dermatology patients, who practice self-application in their homes. The latter group is systematically underdosed. This is a fundamental problem in the translation of results obtained in formal drug studies run with GCP into topical drug application and clinical efficacy when the same substances or products are applied at home. Home treatment may easily be less efficient not only due to poor adherence but also for technical reasons related to the application of the product to skin afflicted with disease. Variation of application and applied dose is in any case high and may easily invalidate dose-finding studies when, for example, dose escalations 1 %, 2.2 %, and 5 % are compared. Variation of dose for technical reasons is a paramount problem of topical therapy in dermatology, setting narrow limits for what can be achieved with topical medicines in practical use by patients treating themselves at home for months.

8.5   Patient Education and Training Using a Fluorescent Test Cream and Supervised Application Can Reduce the Variation of Application

A fluorescent cream was successfully used for the training of patients with hand dermatitis [8]. A similar fluorescent cream was used for the whole body to demonstrate skin fields that were neglected or treated irregularly with a cream as described above [9]. The same group defined a concept named "The Fluorescent-cream Educational Session (FES)" applicable to any body site and every skin disease. The concept included a period of self-practice followed by a second examination. Using the FES neglected areas were reduced from 29 % at the baseline visit to 13.6 % at the follow-up visit 2 weeks later where the treated areas also had been treated more evenly. The mean time for application at the baseline visit was 2.7 min and 3.9 min at the follow-up visit 2 weeks later. Thus, there is a valid training instrument of documented efficacy ready for use in the clinic and as a training session before a pharmaceutical study is started.

8.6   Conclusion

This review highlights the unpleasant fact of high variability of topical drug application simply for technical reasons and independent of other factors determining adherence to treatment. Even in controlled GCP studies with adherent participants, who are motivated and in good general health physically and mentally, variation is major. This should influence industry's designing of dose-finding studies using topical drugs. Dose-escalation studies on topical drugs shall be based on a sample size calculation that realistically takes the huge variation of application by study participants despite good will into consideration, which means that samples have to be sufficiently large in comparative studies to depict a difference of an active product formulated in different and rather close percentages. In dermatological practice with so many confounders, the variation of topical drug application for technical reasons simply related to patient's application is even higher and is likely a common reason for local treatment failures. Intensified patient instruction in correct application of the topical product is only exceptionally practiced in busy routine. To determine what kind of dose (underdose, overdose, or correct dose) patients are using, the

Medication Event Monitoring System (MEMS) is the most reliable device and considered the gold standard for monitoring medication adherence [10]. MEMS can document the actual used dose by recording the time at which medication tubes are opened. However, they are costly devices and not practical in contrast to self-reported measures which are inexpensive and easy to use. A patient training course using a fluorescent test cream and supervised application and with follow-up was introduced and documented efficient but seemingly neglected by dermatologist and dermatology nurses despite the obvious rationale of such approach in improving outcome of local treatment.

References

1. Schlagel CA, Sanborn EC (1964) The weights of topical preparations required for total and partial body injunction. J Invest Dermatol 42:253–256
2. Long CC, Finlay AY (1991) The finger-tip unit—a new practical measure. Clin Exp Dermatol 16:444–447
3. Ivens UI, Steinkjer B, Serup J, Tetens V (2001) Ointment is evenly spread on the skin, in contrast to creams and solutions. Br J Dermatol 145:264–267
4. Ulff E, Maroti M, Kettis-Lindblad A, Kjellgren KI, Ahlner J, Ring L, Serup J (2007) Single application of a fluorescent test cream by healthy volunteers: assessment of treated and neglected body sites. Br J Dermatol 156:974–978
5. Vind-Kezunovic D, Serup J (2016) Variation of topical application to skin under good clinical practice (GCP): a "best performance" scenario. J Dermatol Treat Review 12:1–3
6. Stenberg C, Larkö O (1985) Sunscreen application and its importance for the sun protection factor. Arch Dermatol 121:1400–1402
7. Storm A, Benfeldt E, Andersen SE, Serup J (2008) A prospective study of patient adherence to topical treatments: 95% underdose. J Am Acad Dermatol 59:975–980
8. Bankova L, Lindenau S, Fuchs S, Tittenbach J, Fischer TW, Elsner P (2002) Influence of the galenic form of skin-protective preparation on the application pattern assessed by a fluorescence method. Exog Dermatol 1:313–318
9. Ulff E, Maroti M, Serup J (2013) Fluorescent cream used as an educational intervention to improve the effectiveness of self-application by patients with atopic dermatitis. J Dermatol Treat 24:268–271
10. Greenlaw SM, Yentzer BA, O'Neill JL, Balkrishnan R, Feldman SR (2010) Assessing adherence to dermatology treatments: a review of self-report and electronic measures. Skin Res Technol 16:253–258

Part III
Adherence in Specific Diseases

Chapter 9
Adherence in Acne

Scott A. Davis, Xi Tan, Stephanie Snyder, Ian Crandell, Amir Al-Dabagh, Hsien-Chang Lin, Rajesh Balkrishnan, Jongwha Chang, and Steven R. Feldman

Adapted with permission of the *American Journal of Clinical Dermatology* from:
Tan X, Al-Dabagh A, Davis SA, et al. Medication Adherence, Healthcare Costs and Utilization Associated with Acne Drugs in Medicaid Enrollees with Acne Vulgaris. *Am J Clin Dermatol.* 2013; 14:243–251.
and
Snyder S, Crandell I, Davis SA, Feldman SR. Medical Adherence to Acne Therapy: A Systematic Review. *Am J Clin Dermatol.* 2014; 15:87–94.

S.A. Davis (✉)
Department of Dermatology, Wake Forest School of Medicine, Winston-Salem, NC, USA

Division of Pharmaceutical Outcomes and Policy, University of North Carolina Eshelman School of Pharmacy, Chapel Hill, NC, USA
e-mail: sdavis81@email.unc.edu

X. Tan • R. Balkrishnan
Department of Clinical, Social and Administrative Sciences, College of Pharmacy, University of Michigan, Ann Arbor, MI, USA

S. Snyder • I. Crandell • A. Al-Dabagh
Department of Dermatology, Wake Forest School of Medicine, Winston-Salem, NC, USA

H.-C. Lin
School of Public Health, Indiana University, Bloomington, IN, USA

J. Chang
Division of Health Services Research, Department of Public Health Sciences, College of Medicine, Pennsylvania State University, Hershey, PA, USA

S.R. Feldman
Departments of Dermatology, Pathology, and Public Health Sciences, Wake Forest School of Medicine, Winston-Salem, NC, USA

© Springer International Publishing Switzerland 2016   77
S.A. Davis (ed.), *Adherence in Dermatology*,
DOI 10.1007/978-3-319-30994-1_9

9.1   Introduction

Poor adherence is a common cause for treatment failure in treatable diseases such as acne. Numerous studies have examined this relationship, along with the reasons why patients tend to not adhere to their acne medications and methods that may improve their adherence. Poor adherence can include failure to obtain the medication, "drug holidays," early discontinuation, or simply misunderstanding how the medication is supposed to be used. Insufficient adherence leads to the addition of unnecessary acne treatments, patient frustration and dissatisfaction, and increase in medical expense. Only about 50 % of patients may adhere properly to the therapeutic regimen defined by their dermatologist [1, 2].

In a meta-analysis performed by McDonald et al. [3], as many as 17 studies showed a statistically significant relationship between medication adherence and improved efficacy. Hence, for a medication to work properly, it must be taken regularly and correctly, and a better understanding of this relationship is crucial to improving therapeutic success rates. First, examining the methods used to measure such relationships must be analyzed so that the differences between methodologies and the data collected from these studies can be taken into account. Then, the reasons behind poor adherence can be examined, so that, ultimately, strategies for enhancing adherence can be devised. The purpose of this study is to examine patient adherence to prescribed acne medications, compare available adherence data, and investigate the factors that affect adherence. We close with some practical tips that physicians can use to improve adherence in their acne patients.

9.2   Methods

For this study, we performed an analysis of data from the MarketScan Medicaid Database, followed by a systematic review of the literature.

9.2.1   MarketScan Analysis: Study Design, Data Source, and Study Population

This is a retrospective cohort study from January 1, 2004, to December 31, 2007, using the MarketScan Medicaid Database, which contains administrative claims data for Medicaid enrollees from eight states across the USA. The database is completely compliant with the Health Insurance Portability and Accountability Act (HIPAA), and all data involved are de-identified. The data cover both fee-for-service (FFS) and managed care plans. This study focused on the initial treatment phase; thus, the index date was defined as the date on which a prescription for an acne-related drug was first filled. The index period began on July 1, 2004, following the 6-month pre-index period (washout period), and ended on July 1, 2007, after which there was a 6-month post-index period. Given the general clinical course of acne and the time required for treatment to take effect, the follow-up period was set as 90 days after the index date, and all outcome measures and analyses were based on the 90-day follow-up period unless otherwise specified.

Individuals who had at least one medical claim for a diagnosis of acne based on the International Classification of Diseases, Ninth Revision, Clinical Modification (ICD-9-CM) code 706.1 were included in the study. Other inclusion criteria were as follows: (1) aged 0–64 years on the index date, (2) continuously enrolled in Medicaid during the study period, and (3) had at least one drug claim for acne-related medications during the index period. The exclusion criteria were as follows: (1) Medicaid and Medicare dual eligibility (since the dataset may not have detailed claims for these dual eligible individuals), (2) had the first acne prescription filled before July 1, 2004, and after July 1, 2007, and (3) had data quality issues (e.g., a patient who was coded for more than one birth year, gender, or race category).

9.2.2 Measurements and Outcomes: Medication Adherence and Treatment-Associated Measures

Acne medication adherence was the primary outcome we measured. We measured adherence using medication possession ratio (MPR), which is the ratio of the number of days for which medication was dispensed divided by the number of days for which medication was needed [4]. This method assumed that, if a prescription was filled, the drugs were taken or applied. We evaluated each patient's adherence rate during the 90 days following the index date, truncating the MPR into the range between 0 and 1. We categorized MPRs ≥0.8 as adherent and MPRs <0.8 as not adherent.

We calculated the MPRs for each acne drug class and a composite MPR as a measure of adherence to any acne-related drug. Acne-related drugs were categorized into different drug classes: oral antibiotics, topical antibiotics, injectable antibiotics, oral retinoids (oral isotretinoin), topical retinoids, oral contraceptives, antifungal agents, antiviral agents, oral glucocorticoids, topical glucocorticoids, injectable glucocorticoids, glucocorticoid powders, vitamins, and others. "Others" included benzoyl peroxide products, azelaic acid, and salicylic acid. We classified fixed-dose combination medication into the drug classes of the active ingredients. We established indicators of whether the drugs in each drug class were ever used and summed the number of acne drug classes used per patient. We also calculated total refill numbers for each patient during the 90-day follow-up period and created a dummy variable indicating whether or not a patient had a refill.

9.2.3 Health Utilization and Costs

We used acne-related outpatient visits, as identified by ICD-9-CM classification code 706.1, to measure health utilization. We counted the total number of acne-related outpatient visits within the 90-day follow-up period for each patient and also created a dummy variable indicating whether a patient had an acne-related outpatient visit. The cost evaluation took a third-party payer perspective; thus, we used reimbursements made by Medicaid. We computed both acne-related drug costs and outpatient visit costs for each patient during the 90-day follow-up period. Total acne-related healthcare costs were the sum of drug costs and outpatient visit costs during the same follow-up period.

9.2.4   Other Variables

We used the Charlson Comorbidity Index (CCI) to measure the number and severity of comorbidities as a summary of overall disease burden [5]. The index assigned the weights (1, 2, 3, 6) to several major diseases to represent the severity of these conditions. The higher the CCI score, the more severe the comorbidities the patient had. We computed the CCI score for each patient during the pre-index period. Other independent variables were patient characteristics such as age, race, and gender.

9.2.5   Statistical Analyses

The unit of analysis was the individual patient. We conducted descriptive analyses, presented as mean (standard deviation) or percentage, for all outcome variables and patient characteristics. We performed MPR calculations for the use of any acne-related drug, for the use of each acne drug class, for the subgroup with drug refills, and for the subgroup without drug refills. We also identified the proportion of patients who were adherent (MPR ≥ 0.8) in each specific subgroup. We utilized a logistic regression to assess the predictors of acne medication adherence. The independent variables comprised patient characteristics, CCI score, refill indicator, and indicators of drug used. We also tested the effect of number of acne drug classes used on adherence using a logistic regression. Moreover, we examined the factors associated with whether or not a patient got a refill using a logistic regression. The potential predictors included in the model were patient characteristics, CCI score, and the indicators of drug used.

In addition, we assessed the associations of medication adherence with health utilization and costs, after controlling for patient and treatment characteristics. In terms of acne-related outpatient visits, we conducted both logistic regression and negative binomial regression. We chose the negative binomial regression rather than the Poisson regression due to the overdispersion of the data. The multivariate linear regression of original total acne-related healthcare costs violated the normality and homoscedasticity assumptions. Instead, we used natural log transformed costs as the dependent variable and applied robust variance estimation in the multivariate linear model. We conducted all statistical analyses using Stata™ 12 (Stata Corp LP, TX, USA) [6]. The level of statistical significance was 5 %.

9.2.6 Systematic Review

A MEDLINE search was performed for randomized controlled trials published between 1978 and June 2013, focusing on patient adherence to prescribed acne medications (Fig. 9.1). The search was limited to English-language full-text randomized controlled trials that contained the keywords "compliance" or "adherence," and "acne." This yielded 122 results. We excluded studies of physician adherence to guidelines, case reports, adherence to medications other than those treating acne, acne treatment efficacy, recommendations for improvement of adherence, and patient behavioral modifications or follow-up appointment attendance. The latter two exclusion criteria were used to more closely reveal medication adherence rather than adherence to lifestyle interventions. Studies that examined adherence to prescribed daily medications—topical, oral, or combination regimens—were included. Of the initial yield of 122 results, 14 met criteria for inclusion in the analysis. Variations were found in the modalities of adherence measurement, factors determining adherence, and criteria for what was to be defined as adherence.

In an attempt to compare topical medication adherence and oral medication adherence, a collective analysis was performed by categorizing adherence numbers into "adherent" and "nonadherent," and these data were evaluated utilizing a test for equality of proportions. For studies with more than two levels of adherence, "adherent" was taken to be the strongest level of adherence examined, and all lower levels of adherence were grouped into "nonadherent." Studies quantifying adherence in different ways (such as percentage of medication taken) were not included in this collective analysis. Included studies with oral adherence data were Miyachi et al. [7], Mufleh et al. [8], Flanders and McNamara [9], Pawin et al. [10], and Marazzi et al. [11]. Included studies with topical adherence data were Miyachi et al. [7], Dréno et al. [2], Pawin et al. [10], Tan et al. [12], Eichenfield et al. [13], Jones-Caballero et al. [14], Baker et al. [15], Marazzi et al. [11], and Cunliffe et al. [16].

9.3 Results

9.3.1 MarketScan Analysis

A total of 24,438 eligible patients were included in this study (Table 9.1). The majority of patients (89.39 %) were aged less than 18 years when they received their first acne-related drugs. The majority of our study population was female (55.63 %) and black (49.76 %). The mean CCI score was only 0.31, suggesting a minor comorbidity burden in our young acne population. About 15 % of the cohort had at least one acne-related drug refill. The average number of acne drug classes per patient was about 2.3. The acne-related drugs most used included oral antibiotics (82.04 %), topical antibiotics (52.65 %), topical retinoids (29.31 %), oral contraceptives (11.74 %), and others (44.93 %). 1.26 % of the population used oral isotretinoin.

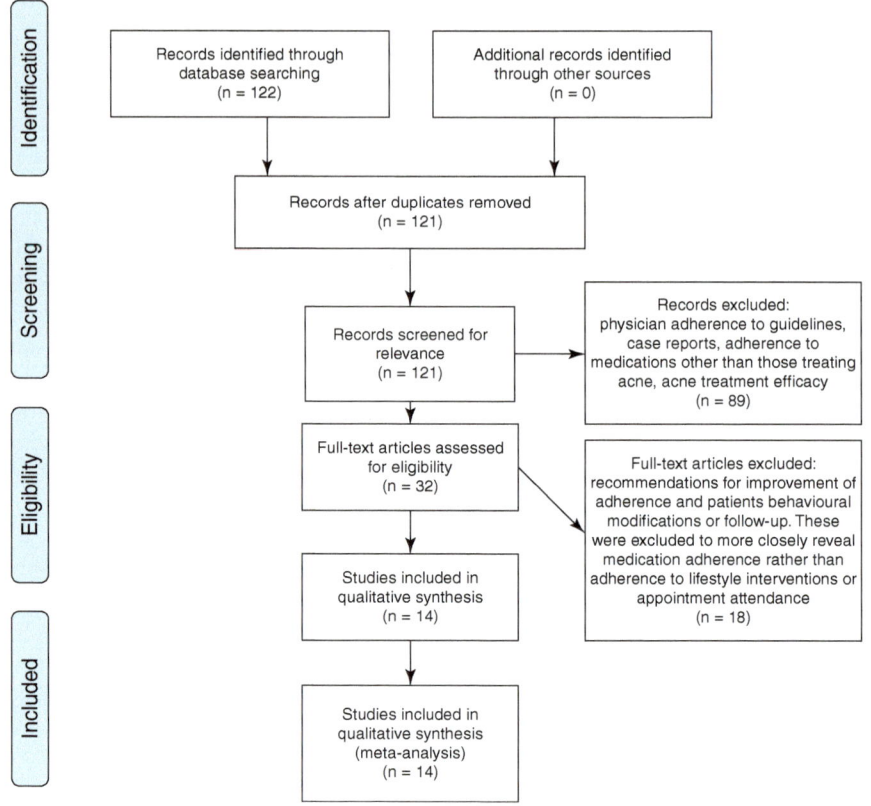

Fig. 9.1 PRISMA 2009 flow diagram

Table 9.2 summarizes the statistics for acne medication adherence. The average adherence rate, as measured by a composite MPR, was 0.34, and only 11.74 % of the patients were categorized as adherent. Patients with drug refills had a much higher adherence rate (MPR = 0.74) than those without refills (MPR = 0.27). The adherence was higher for the use of oral isotretinoin (MPR = 0.78, 57.28 % adherent) and oral contraceptives (MPR = 0.69, 48.99 % adherent) compared with other drug classes. The average adherence rate for topical agents was quite low, approximately 0.30–0.35. The mean MPR for oral antibiotics (0.21) was relatively low as well.

Table 9.3 illustrates the results of the logistic regression examining the predictors of acne medication adherence. As age increased, the likelihood of adherence increased. Black patients were less likely than their white counterparts to be adherent (odds ratio [OR] = 0.82, $p < 0.001$). For every unit of increase in the CCI score, the odds of adherence to acne drugs decreased by a factor of 0.84 ($p < 0.001$). Male patients had a 20 % higher odds of adherence than female patients ($p = 0.002$). Having refills was associated with a much higher likelihood

Table 9.1 Descriptive statistics (*N* = 24,438)

	% or mean (SD)
Age, %	
0–17 year	89.39 %
18–25 year	6.13 %
26–49 year	4.13 %
50–64 year	0.35 %
Sex, %	
Male	44.37 %
Female	55.63 %
Race, %	
White	41.37 %
Black	49.76 %
Hispanic	2.70 %
Other	6.17 %
Charlson Comorbidity Index	0.31 (0.70)
Refill indicator (yes/no)[a]	0.15 (0.36)
Number of acne drug classes used	2.34 (1.17)
Use of acne drugs, %	
Topical antibiotics	52.65 %
Oral antibiotics	82.04 %
Injectable antibiotics	2.29 %
Topical retinoids	29.31 %
Oral retinoids	1.26 %
Oral contraceptives	11.74 %
Topical glucocorticoids	9.31 %
Oral glucocorticoids	0.50 %
Injectable glucocorticoids	0.00 %
Glucocorticoid powders	0.00 %
Antifungal agents	0.12 %
Antiviral agents	0.00 %
Vitamins	0.00 %
Others	44.93 %
Healthcare utilization	
Acne-related outpatient visits during the 90-day follow-up period	0.52 (1.16)
Healthcare costs	
Acne-related drug costs during the 90-day follow-up period	85.16 (109.11)
Acne-related outpatient visit costs during the 90-day follow-up period	22.86 (47.90)
Acne-related total healthcare costs during the 90-day follow-up period	108.02 (133.85)

[a]With ≥1 drug refills

Table 9.2 Medication adherence

	Medication possession ratio (MPR) [mean (SD)]	Adherent patients[a] [n (%)][b]
All acne patients with any acne-related medications	0.34 (0.30)	2868 (11.74%)
Patients with drug refills	0.27 (0.23)	1000 (4.80%)
Patients without drug refills	0.74 (0.29)	1868 (51.57%)
Adherence to different acne drug classes		
Topical antibiotics	0.33 (0.20)	501 (3.89%)
Oral antibiotics	0.21 (0.22)	809 (4.04%)
Injectable antibiotics	0.10 (0.05)	0 (0.00%)
Topical retinoids	0.31 (0.18)	164 (2.29%)
Oral retinoids	0.78 (0.27)	177 (57.28%)
Oral contraceptives	0.69 (0.30)	1406 (48.99%)
Topical glucocorticoids	0.30 (0.17)	45 (1.98%)
Oral glucocorticoids	0.30 (0.17)	2 (1.64%)
Antifungal agents	0.30 (0.20)	1 (3.33%)
Others	0.35 (0.20)	461 (4.20%)

[a]Adherence if MPR ≥0.8, nonadherence if MPR <0.8
[b]The denominator of the percentage was the number of patients who were in the specific subgroup

of adherence (OR = 19.07, $p < 0.001$). In another logistic regression model, we found that one additional drug class increased the odds of being adherent about twice (OR = 2.02, $p < 0.001$), after controlling for age, race, gender, comorbidity, and drug refills.

Table 9.4 displays the factors associated with acne drug refills. Being older, male, white, and having less severe comorbidities were all associated with high odds of getting an acne drug refill. The likelihood of getting a drug refill was also associated with the type of drug used: using topical antibiotics, topical retinoids, oral retinoids, oral contraceptives, and antifungal agents increased the odds, while using oral antibiotics decreased the likelihood.

Table 9.5 shows the results from the logistic regression of acne-related outpatient visits, the negative binomial regression of acne-related outpatient visits, and the multivariate linear regression of total acne-related healthcare costs with robust standard errors. Adherence was a strong predictor for acne-related outpatient visit and healthcare costs. Adherent patients had approximately 2.7 times more acne-related outpatient visits ($p < 0.001$) and 3.5 times greater acne-related healthcare costs ($p < 0.001$), relative to those who were not adherent. Age and gender were not significant factors associated with acne-related outpatient visits or costs. Black and Hispanic patients had 16% more acne-related outpatient visits than whites. Patients with more severe comorbidities had fewer acne-related outpatient visits ($p < 0.001$). Getting an acne drug refill was associated with only a 7% increase in the number of outpatient visits ($p = 0.049$) and a 62% increase in total healthcare costs ($p < 0.001$). After controlling for medication use behavior, patients prescribed with

Table 9.3 Predictors of acne medication adherence (yes/no) using logistic regression (*N*=24,438)

Independent variables	Dependent variable: acne medication adherence (yes/no) odds ratio (95 % CI)
Age group	
0–17 year	Reference
18–25 year	1.61 (1.34, 1.93)**
26–49 year	1.88 (1.49, 2.37)**
50–64 year	3.02 (1.18, 7.73)*
Race	
White	Reference
Black	0.82 (0.74, 0.91)**
Hispanic	1.03 (0.76, 1.38)
Others	0.97 (0.78, 1.19)
Charlson Comorbidity Index	0.84 (0.77, 0.91)**
Gender	
Female	Reference
Male	1.20 (1.07, 1.34)**
Refill indicator(yes/no)	19.07 (17.27, 21.07)**
Use of acne drugs (yes/no)	
Oral antibiotics	1.90 (1.65, 2.18)**
Topical antibiotics	1.61 (1.44, 1.81)**
Injectable antibiotics	0.76 (0.56, 1.05)
Oral retinoids	5.65 (4.18, 7.63)**
Topical retinoids	3.18 (2.88, 3.52)**
Oral contraceptives	3.14 (2.74, 3.59)**
Antifungal agents	4.54 (1.86, 11.07)**
Oral glucocorticoids	2.95 (1.77, 4.91)**
Topical glucocorticoids	1.43 (1.23, 1.67)**
Others	1.71 (1.54, 1.90)**
Intercept	0.008 (0.007, 0.010)**

*$p<0.05$; **$p<0.01$

oral antibiotics had 50.9 % fewer acne-related outpatient visits ($p<0.001$) and 51.7 % lower acne-related total costs ($p<0.001$).

9.3.2 Systematic Review

The analyzed studies used various methods, both subjective and objective, for gathering adherence data. Some used a combination of methods. Each reported adherence values for topical medications, oral medications, and/or a combination of the two (Table 9.6). A collection of risk factors for nonadherence were also extrapolated from the studies.

Table 9.4 Predictors of getting an acne drug fill or not using logistic regression ($N = 24{,}438$)

Independent variables	Dependent variable: refill indicator (yes/no) Odds ratio (95 % CI)
Age group	
0–17 year	Reference
18–25 year	1.57 (1.37, 1.81)**
26–49 year	1.63 (1.36, 1.96)**
50–64 year	1.10 (0.47, 2.56)
Race	
White	Reference
Black	0.69 (0.63, 0.74)**
Hispanic	0.68 (0.54, 0.87)**
Others	0.76 (0.65, 0.89)**
Charlson Comorbidity Index	0.90 (0.85, 0.96)**
Gender	
Female	Reference
Male	1.26 (1.16, 1.37)*
Use of acne drugs (yes/no)	
Oral antibiotics	0.71 (0.65, 0.78)**
Topical antibiotics	1.59 (1.46, 1.74)**
Injectable antibiotics	0.84 (0.66, 1.07)
Oral retinoids	2.38 (1.86, 3.05)**
Topical retinoids	1.67 (1.55, 1.80)**
Oral contraceptives	3.26 (2.94, 3.62)**
Antifungal agents	2.76 (1.29, 5.93)**
Oral glucocorticoids	1.27 (0.79, 2.02)
Topical glucocorticoids	0.99 (0.87, 1.12)
Others	1.38 (1.27, 1.49)**
Intercept	0.11 (0.10, 0.13)**

$*p < 0.05$; $**p < 0.01$

Of the 14 studies, 11 utilized subjective methods of data collection. Miyachi et al. [7] and Dréno et al. [2] measured adherence by assessing the patient's responses to an ECOB (Elaboration d'un outil d'evaluation de l'observance des traitements medicamenteux = Development of a tool for assessment of compliance with drug treatment) self-administered questionnaire versus the expected response validated by the dermatologist's prescription. ECOB is an assessment of a patient's ability to remember four aspects of acne treatment. It has similar questions for topical and oral therapies [2, 7]. Pawin et al. [10] measured adherence similarly, utilizing a dermatologist-directed questionnaire (DDQ). Concordance between adherence and individual questions was tested versus results of the DDQ. Poor adherence was suggested by a patient's inability to name or describe their treatment, or a response implying that the treatment had not been used as directed. Tan et al. [12], Eichenfield et al. [13], Jones-Caballero et al. [14], and Baker et al. [15] collected adherence data by asking patients to rate how

Table 9.5 Predictors of acne-related healthcare utilization and costs ($N = 24{,}438$)

Independent variables	Dependent variables		
	Indicator of acne-related outpatient visit (yes/no)	Number of acne-related outpatient visits	Natural log transformed total healthcare cost
	Odds ratio (95 % CI)[a]	Relative risk (95 % CI)[b]	Coefficients (95 % CI)[c]
Acne medication adherence (yes/no)	4.02 (3.63, 4.46)**	2.75 (2.56, 2.96)**	1.25 (1.18, 1.33)**
Age group			
0–17 year	Reference	Reference	Reference
18–25 year	1.10 (0.97, 1.25)	1.05 (0.94, 1.16)	0.07 (−0.02, 0.16)
26–49 year	0.94 (0.79, 1.11)	0.88 (0.76, 1.00)	−0.07 (−0.18, 0.05)
50–64 year	1.17 (0.65, 2.14)	1.38 (0.88, 2.17)	0.11 (−0.17, 0.39)
Race			
White	Reference	Reference	Reference
Black	1.14 (1.07, 1.22)**	1.16 (1.10, 1.22)**	−0.12 (−0.17, −0.07)**
Hispanic	1.16 (0.96, 1.39)	1.16 (1.00, 1.33)*	0.15 (0.04, 0.26)**
Other	0.93 (0.81, 1.06)	1.02 (0.92, 1.13)	0.02 (−0.07, 0.10)
Charlson Comorbidity Index	0.87 (0.82, 0.91)**	0.90 (0.86, 0.93)**	0.00 (−0.03, 0.04)
Gender			
Female	Reference	Reference	Reference
Male	1.02 (0.95, 1.08)	0.96 (0.91, 1.00)	0.02 (−0.04, 0.07)
Refill indicator (yes/no)	1.24 (1.14, 1.36)**	1.07 (1.00, 1.15)*	0.48 (0.41, 0.56)**
Use of acne drugs (yes/no)			
Oral antibiotics	0.41 (0.38, 0.44)**	0.49 (0.46, 0.52)**	−0.73 (−0.80, −0.66)**
Topical antibiotics	1.67 (1.56, 1.79)**	1.47 (1.39, 1.55)**	0.38 (0.32, 0.44)**
Injectable antibiotics	0.83 (0.66, 1.04)	0.98 (0.82, 1.17)	0.51 (0.36, 0.65)**
Oral retinoids	1.59 (1.24, 2.05)**	2.73 (2.33, 3.19)**	0.59 (0.42, 0.76)**
Topical retinoids	1.72 (1.61, 1.83)**	1.50 (1.43, 1.58)**	0.49 (0.43, 0.54)**
Oral contraceptives	0.67 (0.60, 0.75)**	0.80 (0.73, 0.86)**	0.07 (−0.01, 0.15)
Antifungal agents	2.96 (1.32, 6.64)**	1.36 (0.76, 2.42)	0.32 (0.06, 0.59)*
Oral glucocorticoids	1.03 (0.69, 1.53)	0.99 (0.73, 1.36)	0.59 (0.40, 0.78)**
Topical glucocorticoids	1.18 (1.07, 1.31)**	1.19 (1.11, 1.29)**	0.55 (0.46, 0.63)**
Others	1.42 (1.33, 1.51)**	1.30 (1.23, 1.37)**	0.20 (0.14, 0.26)**
Intercept	0.37 (0.33, 0.41)**	0.41 (0.38, 0.45)**	3.68 (3.59, 3.77)**

$*p < 0.05$; $**p < 0.01$
[a]Logistics regression of acne-related outpatient visit
[b]Negative binomial regression of the numbers of acne-related outpatient visits
[c]Multivariate linear regression of total acne-related healthcare costs, using robust standard errors

often they used their medications as prescribed on either a high to low compliance or usage frequency scale. Other subjective methods included patient interviews, self-monitoring cards, patient diaries, and self-reports [17, 21–25].

Although data collected objectively were in shorter supply, the authors who presented this information allowed for enhanced comprehension beyond what could be drawn from subjective data alone. Aside from the subjective patient interviews, Mufleh et al. [8] also utilized pill counts. Compliance was defined as equal to the number of pills actually used divided by the number of pills that should have been used and multiplied by 100 to give a percentage. Likewise, Zaghloul et al. [17] compared subjective data with that extrapolated from pill counts and topical medication weights. The number of prescriptions filled served as the objective measurement in the trial by Cook-Bolden [18]. Yentzer et al. [19] used a Medication Event Monitoring System cap to allow for an objective way to collect data by recording the date and time when the cap on the medication tube of once-daily benzoyl peroxide was removed.

In a collective analysis of the data (Table 9.6), a test of equality of proportions was performed and showed no significant difference between oral and topical acne medication adherence. The overall oral adherence rate was 76.3 %, and the overall topical adherence rate was 75.8 % ($p=0.927$).

Among the results of these studies, many authors found trends to help predict which patients would be more likely to adhere to treatment regimens. Good adherence correlated with patients who had a better understanding of acne and its treatment [7]. The best adherers used cosmetics, experienced good clinical improvement, had more severe acne, used either isotretinoin or topical therapy alone, and were both knowledgeable about and satisfied with their treatment [2]. An increase in acne disability and decrease in duration of treatment or alcohol intake had a good correlation with high compliance [8]. Topical therapy adherence was positively associated with the negative impact of acne on quality of life [12, 17].

Risk factors for nonadherence were also examined in 7 of the 15 studies assessed (Table 9.7). The occurrence of side effects and young age were both cited as reasons in more than half of these [2, 7, 12, 14, 20]. Forgetfulness was also commonly associated with poor adherence in several studies [2, 12, 14, 17]. Other factors linked to nonadherence included treatment dissatisfaction, a moderate to high Dermatology Life Quality Index (DLQI) score (i.e., severe quality-of-life impact), the use of over-the-counter topical medication or previous systemic therapy, a lack of symptom improvement, a lack of treatment knowledge, male gender, low education level, living alone/single, unemployment, being too busy, frustration, and other comorbidities [2, 7, 8, 12, 17, 20].

9.4   Discussion

Reported adherence values in the systematic review ranged from as low as 7 % to as high as 98 %. An equality of proportions test allowed for a more collective analysis of these values. Although the cumulative values collected from these studies suggest

Table 9.6 Summary of data from 14 studies on acne medication adherence

Study; year; country	Sample size	Oral adherence rate	Topical adherence rate	Measurement methods used	Adherence factors examined
Miyachi et al. [7]; 2011; Japan	428	7 %, 14 % combination oral	52 %, 49 % combination topical	Self/dermatologist questionnaires, ECOB questionnaire	Age, onset age, parental acne, DLQI, PC, other guidance, scarring, improvement in acne
Dréno et al. [2]; Sweden, Denmark, Norway, Spain, Hong Kong, India, Philippines, Singapore, Brazil, Chile, Colombia, Mexico, Venezuela, Canada, USA	3,339	54 % ISO; 46 % combination oral and topical	60 %, 56 % combination oral and topical	Self/dermatologist questionnaires, ECOB questionnaire	Age, occurrence of side effects, improvement in acne, previous systemic therapy, patient education, PCP, DLQI, acne severity, use of cosmetics
Mufleh et al. [8]; 1999; UK	20	89.9 % ± 11.5 (pill-count method); 93.2 % ± 7.6 (interview method)	Not examined	Pill-count method, compliance assessment questionnaire	Acne disability (acne disability index), acne severity (Leeds grading technique), duration of treatment, alcohol intake, level of education, living alone

(continued)

Table 9.6 (continued)

Study; year; country	Sample size	Oral adherence rate	Topical adherence rate	Measurement methods used	Adherence factors examined
Pawin et al. [10]; 2009; France	246	96 % had good adherence; combined oral and topical, 81 % had good adherence to one or both; 59 % had poor adherence	54 % had good adherence; 46 % had poor adherence	Self/dermatologist questionnaire	Treatment modality
Tan et al. [12]; 2009; Canada	152	Not examined	24 % rated as 100 % adherent to therapy; 49 % rated as 75–99 % adherent to therapy; 26 % rated as <75 % adherent to therapy	Questionnaire after 2 months of therapy	Age, gender, duration of acne, education level, third-party drug plan coverage, smoking history, recreational drug use, ingestion of alcohol, number of prescribed topicals, facial acne severity, QoL score
Eichenfield et al. [13]; 2008; USA	544	Not examined	94.5 %, 93.5 %, and 94.5 % at weeks 3, 6, and 12, respectively, for patients using 0.04 % tretinoin gel; 94.7 %, 96.5 %, and 94.6 %, respectively, for patients using 0.1 % tretinoin gel	Questionnaire	
Zaghloul et al. [17]; 2005; UK	403	ISO therapy 71.4 %	Topical and oral medications other than ISO: 35.2 %	The pill-count/weight method	Gender, marital status, age, employment status, treatment distribution, first-time and multi-time ISO treatment, paying for prescription, smoking, alcohol consumption, acne severity, DLQI

	N				Acne severity and initial health beliefs
Flanders and McNamara [9]; 1984; USA	28	49 % overall average		Self-assessment questionnaire	Acne severity and initial health beliefs
Jones-Caballero et al. [14]; 2008; Spain	1,628	Not examined	57.4 % reported "everyday" use; 38.8 % reported "almost everyday" use; 3.5 % reported "sometimes"; 0.4 % reported "almost never"	Self-reported adherence to treatment in which a researcher asked patients how often they had been using the treatment, using a four-item scale (every day, almost every day, sometimes, or almost never)	Gender, QoL, age, employment, lack of time, forgetting, boring treatment, side effects
Baker et al. [15]; 2001; USA	2,545	Not examined	47 % of subjects reported applying medication daily; 45 % applied it almost daily	Self-assessment questionnaire	
Marazzi et al. [11]; 2002; England	188	Not examined	89 % of ISO/erythromycin group and 70 % of benzoyl peroxide/erythromycin group were 76–100 % compliant at each assessment time	Patient diary cards; the study nurse/pharmacist noted on the case report forms whether or not the patients had applied the medication according to the protocol (yes/no)	
Cunliffe et al. [16]; 2005; UK	246	Not examined	Mean adherence rate among patients using clindamycin/zinc gel once daily, 98 %; mean adherence rate using clindamycin/zinc gel twice daily, 92 %; mean adherence using clindamycin gel twice daily, 92 %	Patient diaries	Dosing frequency

(continued)

Table 9.6 (continued)

Study; year; country	Sample size	Oral adherence rate	Topical adherence rate	Measurement methods used	Adherence factors examined
Cook-Bolden [18]; the MORE trial; 2006; USA	1,979	Not examined	Adapalene only at 12 weeks (self-reports), 88.3%; add-on study arms at 12 weeks (self-reports), 87%; adapalene only at 12 weeks (prescription refills), 80.3%; add-on study arms at 12 weeks (prescription refills), 80.4%	Self-reports and prescription refills	Time elapsed since the last appointment
Yentzer et al. [19]; 2009; USA	11	Not examined	82% adherent on day 1; 45% at 6 weeks	Electronic medication event monitoring system	Time elapsed since the last appointment
Tan et al. [20]; 2013; USA	24,438	Antibiotics, 4.04%; retinoids (ISO), 57.28%; contraceptives, 48.99%; glucocorticoids, 1.64%	Antibiotics, 3.89%; retinoids, 2.29%; glucocorticoids, 1.98%	MPR[a]	Age, comorbidity, gender, number of drug refills, and number of drug classes used

DLQI Dermatology Life Quality Index, *ECOB* elaboration d'un outil d'evaluation de l'observance des traitements medicamenteux (development of a tool for assessment of compliance with drug treatment), *ISO* isotretinoin, *MPR* medication possession ratio, *PC* prior consultation, *QoL* quality of life

[a]Ratio of the number of days for which medication was dispensed divided by the number of days for which medication was needed (as determined by days between medication fills)

Table 9.7 Assessment of risk factors for nonadherence

	Miyachi et al. [7]	Dréno et al. [2]	Mufleh et al. [8]	Tan et al. [12]	Zaghloul et al. [17]	Jones-Caballero et al. [14]	Tan et al. [20]
Treatment dissatisfaction	X	X					
DLQI high score	X				X		
Use of OTC medication	X						
Experience of side effect	X	X		X		X	
Previous systemic treatment		X					
Young age		X			X	X	X
Poor improvement		X		X			
Poor knowledge of treatment	X						
Low education level			X				
Living alone/single			X		X		
Forgetfulness				X	X	X	
Male gender					X	X	
Unemployed					X	X	
Self-pay for prescriptions					X		
Frustration					X		
Too busy					X	X	
Other comorbidities							X

DLQI Dermatology Life Quality Index, *OTC* over-the-counter

a majority adherent population, the methodologies used were so weak that little confidence can be placed on these numbers. There was also no significant difference between self-reported adherence to topical versus oral regimens. This is somewhat surprising, as one would expect patients to be less compliant to a more time-consuming regimen, as is the case with topical preparations. However, the scarcity of studies analyzing the oral route of administration limits this test.

In contrast, the MarketScan analysis suggested that the majority of patients were not adherent to either topical or oral medications. There was also a difference between oral therapy adherence values and topical therapy adherence values, showing a better adherence to oral regimens than to topical formulations. The best adherence was seen with oral isotretinoin. The discrepancies between the compiled clinical trials and the database study illustrate how much a larger sample size, different methods of measurement, selection bias, and differing populations (the database study was Medicaid only) could potentially influence results. The results of adherence measurement in clinical trials may not extrapolate to clinical practice. Better adherence in clinical trials than in clinical practice is expected given the effect of office visits on adherence and the greater number of return visits in clinical trial situations [26–28]. This difference may underlie the finding of higher reported adherence in the clinical trials we analyzed compared with the pharmacy database study, which was based on refill rates for ordinary patients rather than for research subjects.

The most common risk factors for nonadherence cited in the literature were the occurrence of side effects and young age. While the side effects of medications cannot be completely eliminated, perhaps patient education and preparation for these side effects, as well as options to help correct them (moisturizers, medication dosage adjustment, etc.), could assist with side effect toleration. However, poor tolerability may not be a major barrier to adherence. Patients may respond well when told that side effects are a sign that the medication is working [25]. Isotretinoin, whose use is nearly universally associated with annoying side effects, is associated with the highest level of adherence among acne treatments. The high adherence rate for users of oral isotretinoin may result from the fact that these patients inherently had more severe acne conditions, and physicians might give those patients more education about the drug and its potential adverse effects. Additionally, these patients had more frequent regular office visits for acne, and more frequent regular office visits could be an effective way of improving adherence in acne patients [26].

Other reported reasons for nonadherence included treatment dissatisfaction, moderate to high impact on quality of life, use of other treatments, poor improvement, lack of knowledge, low education levels, living alone, being male, being unemployed, self-pay for medications, being frustrated with medication, and being too busy [2, 7, 8, 12, 14, 17]. However, the MarketScan analysis actually found that male patients had higher adherence. Quality patient education, reminder systems, and coupons or rebates could help with most of the problems leading to nonadherence. A study performed by Thiboutot et al. shows the positive relationship between adherence and patient education and counseling [29], while Fenerty et al. investigated the role of various reminder systems in adherence enhancement [30]. Regardless of the patient's education level or employment status, a physician's ability to convey medication information is imperative for treatment success and patient satisfaction. Writing down instructions and supplying additional reading material may assist with this. Even the busiest patients might benefit from reminder systems to help keep them on track. In addition to coupons and rebates for more expensive medications, most acne treatments exist in a generic form for patients who find daily administration of their acne prescription too expensive.

9.5 Practical Strategies for Improving Acne Patients' Adherence

Baldwin [31] and Tan et al. [32] summarized the strategies for improving adherence to acne therapies and topical agents. Foremost among these strategies are the maintenance of good doctor-patient relationships, enhanced quality and quantity of office visits, patient education, and the use of fixed-dose combination therapy.

Recent studies evaluated the potential strategies for improving acne medication adherence especially among teenagers. While more strategies are discussed in the last part of this book, here we describe some strategies that may be particularly useful in acne patients.

9.5.1 Combination Products

A small sample randomized controlled trial (RCT) found that adherence to a fixed-combination topical acne drug was significantly higher than the two separate subcomponents after 12 weeks [33]. A once-a-day regimen of the topical combination product induced much better adherence than a regimen of clindamycin in the morning and tretinoin at night. Although in theory some products work better when applied at a particular time of day, regimens requiring medication use at multiple different times each day are too complex for many patients. After experiencing the frustration of forgetting doses for a while, patients may be prepared to give up and discontinue the regimen entirely.

9.5.2 Samples

Although medication samples are controversial, samples can help circumvent the common problem of primary nonadherence, where the patient does not even obtain or take a single dose of the medication. In dermatology and especially acne, samples can be particularly beneficial since using a topical medication is not as simple as taking a pill [34]. Patients are often unsure how much to apply and want to know the feel of the medication to their skin before deciding on a product [34]. Ideally, patients can see some efficacy while using the sample, maximizing the chance that they will fill the prescription.

9.5.3 Office Visits and "Virtual Office Visits"

A pilot RCT found that compared with standard care, more office visits increased adherence while parents' daily reminders did not [26]. Neither did daily phone call reminders nor customized text messages significantly improve adherence [26, 35], yet a weekly Internet-based survey did [36]. These findings could lead to future well-designed interventions to improve acne medication adherence especially in adolescents who consistently demonstrate poor adherence. We suggest that a patient self-reported Internet-based survey, blogs, or health education and promotion via virtual social network platforms could be the future direction to improve acne medication adherence among teenagers, given the features and lifestyles of today's adolescents. However, the online intervention needs to be more than a mere reminder; it needs to serve as a sign of the physician's caring and guidance through the potentially bewildering treatment process.

9.5.4   Side Effects

It might be tempting to assume that medication side effects always have negative effects on adherence. However, actually the amount of irritation that patients experienced in acne clinical trials has shown no association with their dropout rate, suggesting that patients do not experience irritation negatively if they think it is related to symptom improvement [37]. Framing the expected side effect properly can involve telling patients, "You may experience some irritation; that's a sign the treatment is working." Beneficial side effects, such as possible weight loss from the diuretic spironolactone, can also be emphasized. These examples show that the meaning of side effects can be highly subjective, and physicians can greatly influence their patients' interpretation of reality in a way that improves adherence [38].

9.5.5   Preventing Primary Nonadherence

Estimates of the percentage of acne patients who engage in primary nonadherence – not even filling the prescription – range from 10 % [39] to as high as 27 % for filling a complete regimen of acne treatments [40]. In behavioral economics, a default option, where people must make an effort to choose a different option, is chosen much more often than the same option when there is no default [38]. Therefore, any strategy that can make filling the prescription a default option should help prevent primary nonadherence. An early return visit at 1 week forces patients to obtain the medication promptly, rather than allowing them to procrastinate too long. Electronic prescribing may also help [40], perhaps because patients feel embarrassed to have a prescription sent to the pharmacy and then not fill it. At the return visit, the physician can ask questions that will reveal whether the patient is familiar with the medication. If the patient cannot accurately describe what the medication looks like or feels like, primary nonadherence is probably an issue.

9.6   Conclusion

Although much about medication adherence can be drawn from these studies, further research is needed to help enhance understanding to ultimately improve adherence to acne medications. Certainly, more studies utilizing objective means of measurement are necessary, as these are more reliable. Further, a more standardized measurement modality would be ideal so that the factors contributing to nonadherence could remain the focus of the study, rather than the influence of different measurement tools. Perhaps, with continued exploration, the complexity of acne medication adherence will lessen, and an increase in adherence will lead to enhanced medication success and patient satisfaction.

References

1. Ellis RM, Koch LH, McGuire E, Williams JV (2011) Potential barriers to adherence in pediatric dermatology. Pediatr Dermatol 28(3):242–244
2. Dreno B, Thiboutot D, Gollnick H, Finlay AY, Layton A, Leyden JJ et al (2010) Large-scale worldwide observational study of adherence with acne therapy. Int J Dermatol 49(4):448–456
3. McDonald HP, Garg AX, Haynes RB (2002) Interventions to enhance patient adherence to medication prescriptions: scientific review. JAMA 288(22):2868–2879
4. Steiner JF, Koepsell TD, Fihn SD, Inui TS (1988) A general method of compliance assessment using centralized pharmacy records. Description and validation. Med Care 26(8):814–823
5. Charlson ME, Pompei P, Ales KL, MacKenzie CR (1987) A new method of classifying prognostic comorbidity in longitudinal studies: development and validation. J Chronic Dis 40(5):373–383
6. Stata statistical software: release 12 [computer program] (2011) College Station, TX
7. Miyachi Y, Hayashi N, Furukawa F, Akamatsu H, Matsunaga K, Watanabe S et al (2011) Acne management in Japan: study of patient adherence. Dermatology 223(2):174–181
8. Mufleh L, Gonzalez M, Judodihardjo H, Finlay AY (1999) Compliance is high in patients taking oral isotretinoin for acne. Br J Dermatol 141(55 Suppl):87, Ref Type: Abstract
9. Flanders P, McNamara JR (1984) Prediction of compliance with an over-the-counter acne medication. J Psychol 118(1ST Half):31–36
10. Pawin H, Beylot C, Chivot M, Faure M, Poli F, Revuz J et al (2009) Creation of a tool to assess adherence to treatments for acne. Dermatology 218(1):26–32
11. Marazzi P, Boorman GC, Donald AE, Davies HD (2002) Clinical evaluation of double strength isotrexin versus benzamycin in the topical treatment of mild to moderate acne vulgaris. J Dermatolog Treat 13(3):111–117
12. Tan JK, Balagurusamy M, Fung K, Gupta AK, Thomas DR, Sapra S et al (2009) Effect of quality of life impact and clinical severity on adherence to topical acne treatment. J Cutan Med Surg 13(4):204–208
13. Eichenfield LF, Nighland M, Rossi AB, Cook-Bolden F, Grimes P, Fried R et al (2008) Phase 4 study to assess tretinoin pump for the treatment of facial acne. J Drugs Dermatol 7(12):1129–1136
14. Jones-Caballero M, Pedrosa E, Penas PF (2008) Self-reported adherence to treatment and quality of life in mild to moderate acne. Dermatology 217(4):309–314
15. Baker M, Tuley M, Busdiecker FL, Herndon JH Jr, Slayton RM (2001) Adapalene gel 0.1% is effective and well tolerated in acne patients in a dermatology practice setting. Cutis 68(4 Suppl):41–47
16. Cunliffe WJ, Fernandez C, Bojar R, Kanis R, West F (2005) An observer-blind parallel-group, randomized, multicentre clinical and microbiological study of a topical clindamycin/zinc gel and a topical clindamycin lotion in patients with mild/moderate acne. J Dermatolog Treat 16(4):213–218
17. Zaghloul SS, Cunliffe WJ, Goodfield MJ (2005) Objective assessment of compliance with treatments in acne. Br J Dermatol 152(5):1015–1021

18. Cook-Bolden F (2006) Subject preferences for acne treatments containing adapalene gel 0.1%: results of the MORE trial. Cutis 78(1 Suppl):26–33
19. Yentzer BA, Alikhan A, Teuschler H, Williams LL, Tusa M, Fleischer AB Jr et al (2009) An exploratory study of adherence to topical benzoyl peroxide in patients with acne vulgaris. J Am Acad Dermatol 60(5):879–880
20. Tan X, Al-Dabagh A, Davis SA, Lin HC, Balkrishnan R, Chang J et al (2013) Medication adherence, healthcare costs and utilization associated with acne drugs in Medicaid enrollees with acne vulgaris. Am J Clin Dermatol 14(3):243–251
21. Strauss JS, Krowchuk DP, Leyden JJ, Lucky AW, Shalita AR, Siegfried EC et al (2007) Guidelines of care for acne vulgaris management. J Am Acad Dermatol 56(4):651–663
22. Gollnick H, Cunliffe W, Berson D, Dreno B, Finlay A, Leyden JJ et al (2003) Management of acne: a report from a global alliance to improve outcomes in acne. J Am Acad Dermatol 49(1 Suppl):S1–S37
23. Cramer JA, Roy A, Burrell A, Fairchild CJ, Fuldeore MJ, Ollendorf DA et al (2008) Medication compliance and persistence: terminology and definitions. Value Health 11(1):44–47
24. Balkrishnan R, Kulkarni AS, Cayce K, Feldman SR (2006) Predictors of healthcare outcomes and costs related to medication use in patients with acne in the United States. Cutis 77(4):251–255
25. Lott R, Taylor SL, O'Neill JL, Krowchuk DP, Feldman SR (2010) Medication adherence among acne patients: a review. J Cosmet Dermatol 9(2):160–166
26. Yentzer BA, Gosnell AL, Clark AR, Pearce DJ, Balkrishnan R, Camacho F et al (2011) A randomized controlled pilot study of strategies to increase adherence in teenagers with acne vulgaris. J Am Acad Dermatol 64(4):793–795
27. Feldman SR, Camacho FT, Krejci-Manwaring J, Carroll CL, Balkrishnan R (2007) Adherence to topical therapy increases around the time of office visits. J Am Acad Dermatol 57(1):81–83
28. Heaton E, Levender MM, Feldman SR (2013) Timing of office visits can be a powerful tool to improve adherence in the treatment of dermatologic conditions. J Dermatolog Treat 24(2):82–88
29. Thiboutot D, Zaenglein A, Weiss J, Webster G, Calvarese B, Chen D (2008) An aqueous gel fixed combination of clindamycin phosphate 1.2% and benzoyl peroxide 2.5% for the once-daily treatment of moderate to severe acne vulgaris: assessment of efficacy and safety in 2813 patients. J Am Acad Dermatol 59(5):792–800
30. Fenerty SD, West C, Davis SA, Kaplan SG, Feldman SR (2012) The effect of reminder systems on patients' adherence to treatment. Patient Prefer Adherence 6:127–135, Epub;%2012 Feb 10.:127–35
31. Baldwin HE (2006) Tricks for improving compliance with acne therapy. Dermatol Ther 19(4):224–236
32. Tan X, Feldman SR, Chang J, Balkrishnan R (2012) Topical drug delivery systems in dermatology: a review of patient adherence issues. Expert Opin Drug Deliv 9(10):1263–1271
33. Yentzer BA, Ade RA, Fountain JM, Clark AR, Taylor SL, Fleischer AB Jr et al (2010) Simplifying regimens promotes greater adherence and outcomes with topical acne medications: a randomized controlled trial. Cutis 86(2):103–108
34. Sandoval LF, Semble A, Gustafson CJ, Huang KE, Levender MM, Feldman SR (2014) Pilot randomized-control trial to assess the effect product sampling has on adherence using adapalene/benzoyl peroxide gel in acne patients. J Drugs Dermatol 13(2):135–140
35. Boker A, Feetham HJ, Armstrong A, Purcell P, Jacobe H (2012) Do automated text messages increase adherence to acne therapy? Results of a randomized, controlled trial. J Am Acad Dermatol 67(6):1136–1142
36. Yentzer BA, Wood AA, Sagransky MJ, O'Neill JL, Clark AR, Williams LL et al (2011) An internet-based survey and improvement of acne treatment outcomes. Arch Dermatol 147(10):1223–1224
37. Bartlett KB, Davis SA, Feldman SR (2014) Topical antimicrobial acne treatment tolerability: a meaningful factor in treatment adherence? J Am Acad Dermatol 71(3):581–582

38. Davis SA, Feldman SR (2014) An illustrated dictionary of behavioral economics for health-care professionals. CreateSpace, Charleston
39. Storm A, Andersen SE, Benfeldt E, Serup J (2008) One in 3 prescriptions are never redeemed: primary nonadherence in an outpatient clinic. J Am Acad Dermatol 59(1):27–33
40. Anderson KL, Dothard EH, Huang KE, Feldman SR (2015) The frequency of primary non-adherence to acne treatment. JAMA Dermatol 151:623–626

Chapter 10
Psoriasis and Adherence to Therapy: Individual, Treatment-Related and General Factors

Katrina Hutton Carlsen, Adel Olasz, Karen Marie Carlsen, and Jørgen Serup

10.1 Introduction

Psoriasis is a cumbersome chronic skin disease bearing a major impact on quality of life [1–3]. Psoriasis patients were shown to be among the more challenging groups in dermatology with respect to their carefulness and awareness in following an agreed treatment schedule. There is a major potential for improvement, since high non-adherence has been reported frequently in the literature.

Different therapeutic modalities can be complicated for the patient to act in accordance with. Individual factors among patients are important prerequisites for the provider of treatment when the individual treatment strategy is agreed upon with the patient, the mutual aim being to achieve the best possible therapeutic outcome.

How do psoriasis patients perform with their practising of local treatments, oral treatments, biologic treatments and light therapy? What are the predictors of poor adherence to treatment, specifically in psoriasis, and what determines individual performance in the lack of fulfilment of treatment requirements? What interventions can be made when adherence is low? Which failures of performance can be foreseen and prevented in clinical practice?

Both the provider of treatment and the patient have a key responsibility. The provider shall integrate considerations on adherence at any time when a new treatment is instituted and continued.

K. Hutton Carlsen (✉) • J. Serup
Department of Dermatology, Bispebjerg University Hospital,
Bispebjerg Bakke 23, DK-2400 Copenhagen, Denmark
e-mail: Katrinahuttoncarlsen@hotmail.com; joergen.vedelskov.serup@regionh.dk

A. Olasz
Department of Dermatology, University Hospital of Northern Norway, Tromsø, Norway

K.M. Carlsen
Centre for Rheumatology, Rigshospitalet, Copenhagen University Hospital,
Copenhagen, Denmark

© Springer International Publishing Switzerland 2016
S.A. Davis (ed.), *Adherence in Dermatology*,
DOI 10.1007/978-3-319-30994-1_10

In this chapter, we aim to address these critical issues, bearing in mind that adherence to therapy is as important as choice of medication and initiation of therapy.

10.2   Adherence to Local Treatment

Corticosteroids applied as local treatments are commonly used and the first drug of choice in psoriasis treatment. A broad range of products formulated as creams, ointments, gels and solutions are available. The use of a topical product for treatment of psoriasis can give the impression of a simple form of therapy, but the entire procedure – from intention to treat to correct daily-practised therapy – has multiple steps, all of which may fail.

10.2.1   Patients' Perception of Psoriasis as a Disease and the Influence of Anatomical Site

Psoriasis on visible anatomical sites influences patients' perceptions of the disease and their social life more than psoriasis in areas covered with clothes [4]. Some patients, especially youngsters, are heavily burdened and eager to treat, while other patients over time have developed acceptance and learned to live with their scaly disease with regression to a state of laissez-faire. These patients may even terminate treatment despite visible disease and deliberately choose to view themselves as "normal". Development of acceptance of disease and "give up" attitude strongly influences adherence negatively.

In a study on 495 psoriasis patients, attending dermatologists in Italy found 54 % who perceived psoriasis as a disease or pathology while 44 % considered psoriasis as a non-pathological condition (nuisance, complaint, inconvenience or just a "problem") [4]. Among those who recognised having a disease, more than half of the patients (56 %) assessed the disease as moderate, 27 % assessed it as severe and 17 % assessed it as mild. Psoriasis involving the face occurred in 28 % of patients and the severity of psoriasis on this particular site was perceived greater compared to other sites.

10.2.2   Preferences of Local Treatments

Topical psoriasis treatments as opposed to systemic or biologic treatments have been identified with fewer side effects, more rapid onset of action and acceptable efficacy [5]. Thus, topical treatments are considered justified as a first-line treatment of psoriasis.

A recent study on psoriasis patients showed that cream formulations were preferred compared to other formulations, these being more practical, comfortable to apply and less greasy than ointments [4]. Sixty-nine percent considered their topical medication an approved registered drug and not an emollient while 31 % were uncertain. Half of the patients with affected visible skin locations and normally not covered by clothes carried a topical product to work, school, etc., to follow the treatment schedule.

Psoriasis patients considered the following advantages of topical formulations important: moisturising, felt quickly "absorbed", same product available in various formulations, does not bleach or stain, is not greasy or oily, is not sticky or tacky, is long lasting/long acting, is fragrant or odour-free and is easy to apply/simple to use [6].

A questionnaire-based study from Spain, performed by a panel of experts and members of the Psoriasis Group of the Spanish Academy of Dermatology and Venereology, aired similar experiences with psoriasis treatments as mentioned above. Ointments were considered to be less acceptable than creams due to their tendency to cause stains on textiles and due to their oily consistency and less acceptable than lipophilic gels with respect to ease of application and adhesiveness following application [7]. An overview is presented in Table 10.1.

10.2.3 Prescription, Redemption and Underdosage

A study conducted in Bispebjerg University Hospital, Denmark, among 322 dermatological outpatients suffering from psoriasis, eczema, acne and infections, showed that 30.7 % *did not* redeem their prescriptions on newly prescribed medications. In this group, psoriasis patients were the least adherent group with 38 of 86 (44.2 %) not redeeming the prescription (Table 10.2) [8]. Among patients who did redeem their prescriptions at pharmacies, 95 % underdosed and applied only 35 % of the estimated optimal dosage to the area of skin afflicted with disease [9]. The ratio of applied and expected dose of topical treatment is presented in Fig. 10.1.

These findings are in accordance with an additional study on 53 psoriasis patients, showing 40 % to be non-adherent to medication [10]. A review of the literature reveals that psoriasis patients only apply between 35 and 72 % of the recommended dosage during a treatment course ranging from 14 days to 8 weeks and, additionally, the number of daily applications also varied between 50 and 60 % of daily dosage scheduled [9, 11].

Psoriasis severity can vary between a few plaques or virtually cover the entire skin. With a large area affected by psoriasis, local treatment is not a realistic option. A study of dermatological self-treatment included 20 healthy, highly motivated volunteers, willing to treat their skin surface with a fluorescent test cream, barring the head, neck and skin covered by underwear [12]. For all intents and purposes, approximately 31 % of the skin surface treated did not show any signs of fluorescence. The centre of the back, the upper breast, the axilla with surrounding skin, the legs, the feet and particularly the soles were typical neglected sites. The treated sites also proved to be inadequate; fluorescence was very uneven. This illustrates

Table 10.1 Evaluation of topical treatments of psoriasis, reported from Spain by a panel of experts and members of the Psoriasis Group of the Spanish Academy of Dermatology and Venereology. Data are shown as median (interquartile range). The interquartile range is from 1 (strongly disagree) to 7 (strongly agree) (Ref. [7])

Product	No.	Ease of application	Absorbs well	Causes stains	Oily consistency	Smells bad	Pleasant	Causes itching/ burning	Leaves a residue on hands	Application is time consuming
Ointments										
Expert panel	9	2 (2–3)	2 (2–4)	6 (5–6)	6 (5–6)	3 (2–4)	2 (2–3)	2 (2–2)	6 (5–6)	5 (4–6)
Psoriasis group	26	2.5 (2–5)	4 (3–5)	4 (3–5)	5 (5–6)	2 (1–3)	3 (2–4)	2 (2–3)	4 (3–5)	4 (2.2–5)
Creams										
Expert panel	9	4 (4–6)	4 (4–5)	3 (3–5)	4 (3–5)	2 (2–4)	5 (4–5)	2 (2–2)	4 (3–4)	4 (3–4)
Psoriasis group	35	5 (4.6–6)	5 (4–6)	2 (1–3)	2.5 (1–4)	1 (1–2)	5 (2–6)	2 (1–2.75)	2 (1–3)	2 (2–3.75)
Lipophilic gels										
Expert panel	9	5 (5–6)	6 (5–6)	3 (3–4)	3 (2–4)	2 (1–3)	5 (4–6)	2 (1–2)	3 (2–4)	3 (2–3)
Psoriasis group	14	5 (5–6.75)	6 (5–6)	2 (2–3)	3 (2–4)	1 (1–2)	5 (4–6)	2 (1–2)	2 (1.25–3)	2 (2–3.75)
Foams										
Expert panel	9	6 (6–6)	6 (6–7)	1 (1–1)	1 (1–1)	1 (1–2)	5 (5–6)	2 (1–4)	2 (1–2)	2 (1–2)
Psoriasis group	8	6 (6–7)	6.5 (6–7)	2 (1–2.25)	2 (1–2)	1 (1–2)	5 (2.75–6)	2.5 (1–4.25)	1.5 (1–2)	1.5 (1–2.2)
Solutions										
Expert panel	9	6 (5.5–6.5)	6 (6–6.5)	2 (1.5–3)	1.5 (1.5–2)	2 (1–3)	5.5 (4–6)	3 (2–3.5)	2 (1–2)	2 (1–3)
Psoriasis group	11	6 (5–6.5)	6 (5–6)	2 (1.25–3)	2 (1.25–3)	2 (1–3)	6 (2–6)	4 (2–5)	2 (1–2)	2 (2–3)
Emulsions										
Expert panel	9	5 (5–6)	5 (4–6)	3 (2–3)	3 (2–3)	2 (1–4)	5 (4–5)	2 (2–2)	3 (2–3)	3 (3–3)
Psoriasis group	8	7 (6–7)	7 (5.7–7)	1.5 (1–2)	1 (1–2.25)	1 (1–2)	6 (5–6)	1 (1–2)	2 (1–3)	2 (1.7–5)

Table 10.2 Patients who *did not* redeem their prescriptions for treatment of psoriasis compared to other dermatological diseases, reported in a Danish study (*n*=322) (Ref. [8])

Skin disease	Non-adherence by number	Non-adherence by percentage	Median days to redemption
Psoriasis	38 of 86 patients	44.2%	17
Eczema	43 of 137 patients	31.4%	1
Acne	1 of 11 patients	9.1%	0
Infections	5 of 41 patients	12.2%	1

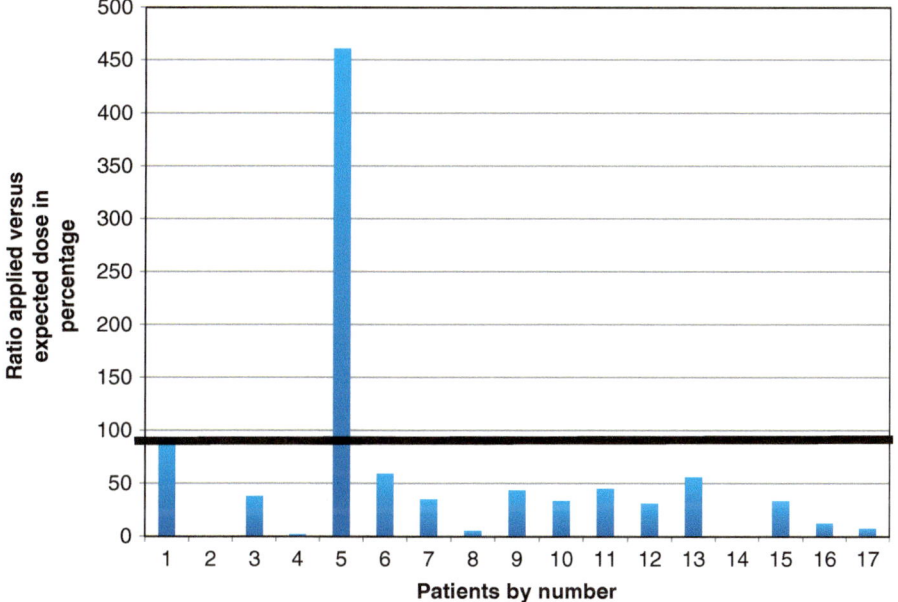

Fig. 10.1 Ratio of de facto applied topical treatment versus expected dose in percentage, reported in a Danish study (*n*=17, patients with psoriasis, eczema, rosacea and lichen planus) (Ref. [9]). Satisfactory adherence rate=100%

the difficulty patients face in applying topical products when exposing a specific site to a constant dose.

Local treatments therefore, generally and by nature, are variable and imprecise. Dosage form depends not only on the chosen topical but also on trivial facts related to treatment discipline, namely, how the product is practically applied by the patient in the home, a task more difficult than hitherto understood. Moreover, the chemical skin barrier in the stratum corneum is very efficient and only allows a small percentage of the applied amount of the active drug to pass into the skin. Only lipophilic molecules smaller than approx. 500 Dalton can pass the skin barrier, distribute and reach the location in the dermis where the particular disease is situated and initiated [13, 14]. It is, therefore, critically important for pharmacological reasons that psoriasis patients are meticulous with their topical applications and are properly informed about this key requirement already at initiation of the treatment. Patient instruction and training in application supervised by a nurse with specialties in dermatology using a fluorescent test cream are efficient educational tools [12, 15].

A study concerning local topical treatments (betamethasone dipropionate cream 0.05 %) has shown that one versus two daily applications had the same clinical effect among eczema patients; however, this result cannot be extrapolated to other diseases [16].

10.2.4 Personal Factors Determining Non-adherence to Topical Treatment

Results from an Italian study with 495 questionnaires sent to dermatology patients showed that patient's explanations for failing to apply or interrupting topical treatment were (average rating from 0 to 5) lack of results within the expected time frame (3.8); inconvenience of therapy (3.7); recognition of an apparently better product (3.7); fear of being subjected to a potentially dangerous product (3.6); excessive cost of the product (3.2); unpleasantness of the product, e.g. greasy or with smell, etc. (3.0); and finally unconvincing attitude of the dermatologist prescribing it (2.5) [4]. Of the respondents, 67 % expected treatment results within 2 weeks of topical usage, while 42 % expected results within 1 week. It appears necessary to reconcile patient's treatment expectations to avoid unnecessary disappointments and early drop out from treatments.

In a study from the USA including 53 psoriasis patients, comparable results were obtained. The main reasons for non-adherence to local topical therapies were frustration with medication efficacy, inconvenience of applications and fear of side effects [10]. In another study from the USA including 193 psoriasis respondents, approximately 50 % of those who did not adhere to prescribed treatments expressed forgetfulness and reported using medication ad hoc after necessity, which, in the majority of cases, should be considered a chaotic treatment schedule [5].

A study of 1281 patients with psoriasis, contacted through the national psoriasis patient associations in France, the UK, Belgium, Germany and the Netherlands, showed that 32 % currently suffered from psoriasis in the face, skinfolds and genital areas. A majority (74 %) considered their psoriasis as moderate or severe; nevertheless, 73 % did not comply with their current treatment. The main reasons for non-adherence were lack of efficacy and messiness of the treatment [17].

10.2.5 Treatment Refusal

Reports of topical treatment refusal have been investigated in 50 psoriasis patients in a study from France [18]. Co-morbidities, localisation of psoriasis on the body and subjective symptoms associated with psoriasis were not significant determinants of refusal. However, comparison of patients who refused treatment with patients who accepted treatment showed that more patients refusing treatment believed psoriasis to be non-manageable (80.0 % versus 61.5 %) and that treatment never works (58.0 % versus 27.5 %). Also, more patients in the treatment refusal group reported some dissatisfaction with their physician [18].

Despite the virtue of local treatment where only the diseased area is treated, there are a large number of limitations and drawbacks. Treatment conditions in homes with cumbersome routine treatment, performed by patients themselves, may often reduce or eliminate their potential to alleviate psoriasis. As mentioned, local treatment of psoriasis is often not used correctly and therefore treatment outcome is unsatisfactory. However, several reasons for poor adherence in psoriasis are reasonable and understandable when viewed in the holistic perspective of life with many responsibilities, needs and priorities competing for awareness.

10.3   Adherence to Oral and Other Systemic Treatments

Patients with moderate and severe psoriasis tend to show higher satisfaction with systemic treatment than to topical treatments [19].

A recent study has rated patients' satisfaction with treatments. Patients were very satisfied with biologic treatments (51.7 %) and other systemic treatments (36.1 %) followed by topical treatments (8.1 %) [20]. Reviewing the range from very dissatisfied, dissatisfied, undecided, satisfied to very satisfied, the overall figure is clearly in disfavour of local treatments accordant with the many limitations of the latter treatment modality as outlined above.

Other studies also showed higher adherence rates to oral treatments versus local topical treatments, indicating that treatment satisfaction and level of adherence accompany each other. A Japanese study of 237 patients with psoriasis showed better adherence to oral treatment than to local treatment, and, surprisingly, only 12.5 % showed high adherence and 32.1 % medium adherence, while as many as 55.4 % showed low adherence [21]. However in the same study, local treatment emerged even worse; 5.6 % showed high adherence, 18.1 % medium adherence and 76.4 % low adherence. Factors significantly influencing adherence to oral systemic treatment were age and annual income. Patients of younger age and patients with low annual income were more inclined to non-adherence. Measurement of adherence by the Morisky Medication Adherence Scale-8 (MMAS-8) confirmed higher adherence to oral treatment with a mean score of 5.2 versus local treatment with a mean score of 4.3 [21].

The status and type of clinics, which may attract different groups of patients, may influence adherence. Notably, more psoriasis patients (90.3 %) visited regional public hospitals once every half-year or more frequently compared to 61.5 % in private clinics and main health-care institutions [21]. Possibly, the latter group suffered psoriasis of milder degree.

In the following text, individual oral medicines used to treat psoriasis will be reviewed to illustrate drug-related pros and cons concerning their use and factors that may influence adherence.

10.3.1 Adherence to Methotrexate

Methotrexate was the first effective systemic drug for psoriasis and continues to be preferential in the treatment of moderate to severe psoriasis [22]. Methotrexate is a cytostatic drug that inhibits the hyperactive mitotic activity of basal cells in the epidermis, considered to be the hallmark of psoriatic disease mechanism. It is prescribed for patients with extensive degree of plaque psoriasis, erythrodermic psoriasis, pustular psoriasis and psoriatic arthritis.

Patients with moderate to severe plaque psoriasis discontinued methotrexate in 41.7 % during a treatment course, mainly due to side effects or lack of response (and fumaric acid ester predominantly in 42.5 %) [23]. Satisfaction with methotrexate and with fumaric acid esters, given as monotherapy under daily life conditions, is comparable for the two drugs [23]. If methotrexate monotherapy is ineffective, the combination of etanercept and methotrexate has been documented to increase the treatment effect on active psoriasis [24].

Psoriatic arthritis may develop after some years of active psoriasis with the need for chronic medication [25]. In a cohort study of 193 patients with psoriatic arthritis, 71 (36 %) stopped their methotrexate treatment with a mean duration of treatment of only 18.6 months [26]. Gastrointestinal complaints were blamed in some cases, although this complaint normally is only experienced initially and often controlled through temporary dose reduction and supplementary treatment with folate. Patients with psoriatic arthritis are alleged to be less responsive to traditional systemic and biologic treatments than patients without arthritis. Effective and sustainable medication for this vulnerable patient group, where complete arthritis clearance is very rarely achieved, is a major challenge [20]. Early diagnosis, early and effective treatment and follow-up consultations are utterly important to enhance patients' objective condition and help their quality of life [27, 28]. Communication between different specialties (e.g. dermatologist and rheumatologist) leads to a more comprehensive treatment approach [25]. Adherence to treatment is especially important in this group, which may be therapy resistant, albeit patients may appreciate a minor reduction of pain as a noteworthy improvement.

10.3.2 Adherence to Fumaric Acid Esters

Fumaric acid esters are chemical compounds from unsaturated dicarbonic acid, reported to be effective in plaque psoriasis, pustular psoriasis and mild psoriatic arthritis [29]. Their use in psoriasis was briefly mentioned above. Psoriasis patients showed high satisfaction (4.17 on a 5-point scale) with fumaric acid esters [20]. However, a retrospective study on fumaric acid ester revealed that 146 of 249 patients (59 %) discontinued their treatment due to lack of efficacy (40 %) and gastrointestinal symptoms (27 %), which are similar results to methotrexate [30]. A lower maintenance dose of fumaric acid ester, less than 240 mg daily, was shown to maintain control of psoriasis in 26 (10 %) patients. A lower dose may reduce gastrointestinal side effects. Fumaric acid esters have a 4-year drug survival rate of 60 % compared to etanercept and adalimumab (40 %) and infliximab (70 %) [30]. Doctors' careful monitoring of disease and treatment balancing therapeutic efficiency versus side effects is, obviously, a critical factor in maintaining psoriasis patients adherence to oral treatment during long-term therapy.

10.3.3   Adherence to Acitretin

Acitretin is a vitamin A analog belonging to the chemical class retinoids, chemicals that reduce hyperproliferation and normalises dyskeratinisation in psoriatic plaques. Psoriasis patients being responders to acitretin treatment express their high satisfaction with acitretin [20]. However, treatment may be followed by dose-dependent adverse effects with signs of hypervitaminosis A, and acitretin treatment maintenance rates are reported low (22.6 %) [20]. Acitretin is generally considered less efficient for plaque psoriasis than other systemic medications, but it may be suitable for treating palmoplantar psoriasis and palmoplantar pustulosis [20]. Adherence is individual and influenced by doctor's monitoring of disease and treatment to maintain an acceptable balance between improvement of disease and the burden of adverse effects.

10.3.4   Adherence to Cyclosporine

Cyclosporine, an immune modulator, was studied in 112 patients treated for 12 weeks [31]. Mean dose of cyclosporine was 2.88 ± 0.74 mg/kg/day. Psoriasis severity decreased by 65.9 % as a mean and quality of life improved by 70.2 %. At 12 weeks, 64.3 % of patients continued treatment beyond the study period, mean dose during maintenance 2.51 ± 0.91 mg/kg/day. Various mild side effects were reported (36.0 %), and "only" 14 % discontinued treatment due to side effects [31]. Patients showed high satisfaction with cyclosporine. Satisfaction was influenced negatively among patients living alone but influenced positively among patients who noted improvement of disease with less flares. The main reason for terminating treatment with cyclosporine appears to be doctor's concern of renal complication and arterial hypertension rather than patient's concern or non-adherence [31].

10.4 Adherence to Biologic Treatment

Biologic agents or biologics are systemic treatments of psoriasis, which have different targets: tumour necrosis factor inhibitors (etanercept (Enbrel®), adalimumab (Humira®) and infliximab (Remicade®, Remsima®, Inflectra®)) and monoclonal antibodies directed against IL-12 and IL-23 (ustekinumab (Stelara®)). Biologics are the most expensive treatments and, therefore, reserved for moderate to severely burdened patients selected according to strict guidelines including recommendations concerning *pretreatment*, *during treatment* and *post-treatment* [32]. Biologics are administered subcutaneously or intravenously at different intervals depending on the product. They may be injected in the prescribing doctor's office and in a hospital outpatient clinic or administered at home by patients themselves after having received training in subcutaneous injection technique.

Studies have shown that patients with psoriasis receiving injections or infusions with biologics have the highest treatment satisfaction with high efficacy and few adverse effects [33–38]. Adherence to biologics is therefore higher compared to other treatments of psoriasis [37, 38]. Despite the generally high level of adherence in patients using biologics, minor differences among the products with respect to adherence appear.

A retrospective unpublished study, from the dermatology department at Bispebjerg University Hospital, Denmark, showed remarkably high primary adherence during treatment with the biologic efalizumab (Raptiva®). In total, 43 patients treated with this biologic and 43 patients treated with TL-01 UV-B light during the same period and in the same ambulatory unit were enrolled and studied consecutively. The groups were comparable with respect to severity of psoriasis according to PASI score, age and gender. The study showed that 0 % of the patients in the biologic group were primary non-adherent during the first 12 weeks of treatment (see Table 10.3). In comparison, 30.2 % of the patients in the TL-01 UV-B light group were non-adherent. However, efalizumab is no longer available, withdrawn by the manufacturer because of a rare neurologic complication.

A prospective case note review including 58 patients, who in total received 84 treatment courses with the biologics etanercept (Enbrel®) (21 treatments), adalimumab (Humira®) (24 treatments), infliximab (Remicade®, Remsima®, Inflectra®) (14 treatments) and ustekinumab (Stelara®) (25 treatments), showed that ustekinumab had the highest long-term adherence, with approximately 90 % of patients remaining on treatment after almost 3 years [39]. Patients treated with ustekinumab were 6.7-fold less likely to withdraw from treatment than patients treated with etanercept. The explanation could possibly be that ustekinumab is administered every 12th week compared to infliximab every 8th week, adalimumab every 2nd week and etanercept once a week [40].

A study has examined 426 psoriasis patient experiences with biologic treatment (adalimumab, etanercept, ustekinumab) grouped as 263 biologic-experienced patients and 163 biologic-naïve patients [41]. The most frequently chosen drug dosing option (38.8 % of all participating patients) was every 2–3 months; 37.3 % chose

Table 10.3 Non-adherence to the biologic efalizumab (Raptiva®) versus narrowband UV-B treatment offered by the outpatient clinic of the Dept. of Dermatology, Bispebjerg University Hospital, Denmark. Days off due to closure of the clinic on holidays, etc., were not included in the results

	Patients	Patients missing >20% of treatments (%)	Patients missing >10% of treatments (%)
Efalizumab			
Men	25	0 (0%)	1 (4%)
Women	18	0 (0%)	0 (0%)
Total	43	0 (0%)	1 (2.3%)
TL-01 UV-B			
Men	25	9 (36%)	15 (60%)
Women	18	4 (22.2%)	11 (61.1%)
Total	43	13 (30.2%)	26 (60.5%)

once every 1–2 weeks. Significant differences were found in the percentage of biologic-naïve patients choosing 2- to 3-month (49.7%) over 1- to 2-week (20.9%) dosing ($P=0.001$). Among biologic-experienced patients, there were no significant findings [41]. The two preferred week-specific intervals chosen by biologic-naïve patients were 12 + weeks (42.3%) and 4 weeks (15.6%). The biologic-experienced patients preferred 12 + weeks (31.2%) and 1 week (25.9%). Thus, dosage interval is also an evolving factor when attempting higher adherence levels, even though the authors did not highlight differences between adalimumab, etanercept and ustekinumab.

Patients offered biologic treatment, often and as part of the qualification for expensive biologics, have tried many different therapies and experienced therapeutic failures. These patients, in particular, may appreciate long-term treatment with biologics providing long-term disease control, a treatment often honoured with high adherence. A new challenge also influencing adherence is educating patients in self-administration as physicians do for insulin in diabetic patients. While learning self-administration technique can be demanding for the patient, it is conceivable that the convenience of not being dependent on professional assistance is compensation enough.

10.5   Adherence to Phototherapy

Phototherapy is often mentioned among first-line treatments offered to patients with advanced psoriasis covering major parts of the skin integument. Ideally, phototherapy should be provided 7 days a week since lymphocytes exert their constant stimulus and keratinocytes proliferate and become dysmature every hour and every day building up the psoriatic plaque. Dosing light and dosing medication daily are, in principle, similar requirements for treatment to show highest effect. Standard approach to administer phototherapy is to provide the treatments in special light therapy units in hospital clinics and private offices. Patients' self-administered phototherapy in their homes, using typically more primitive lamps, is also an option.

Phototherapy provided by clinics and offices has the inbuilt practical limitation that therapy is only accessible within opening hours and not on weekends, holidays, etc., hereby reducing weekly dose. There is also the inconvenience patients have to take time off from work to attend the clinic. Only few clinics have organised special day-care units and flexible drop in systems. The mentioned restrictions limit the performance of phototherapy and motivates disorganisation, irregularity and, in the end, non-adherence to phototherapy.

A recent study assessed adherence to phototherapy in patients with psoriasis and vitiligo [42]. Psoriasis patients were considered adherent if they had attended a minimum of 20 treatment sessions, twice weekly. Of the 851 patients with psoriasis (479 women and 372 men), 53 % received fewer than 20 treatments and approximately one third received fewer than 10 treatment sessions. As an effective treatment, these results should be considered incomplete and inconclusive. Age was the strongest factor in determining adherence to phototherapy. Patients older than 40 years were 1.65 times more inclined to receive 20 or more treatments than the younger age groups. Of the 106 patients with vitiligo, 61 % of patients received 60 or more treatments. Similarly to patients with psoriasis, age was the most important demographic factor influencing adherence.

A small study has been published on patients' adherence to self-administered phototherapy in their homes, compared to oral medication with acitretin [43]. The study included 22 patients receiving acitretin and 16 patients treated with narrowband ultraviolet B at home. Patients were treated with 10–25 mg of acitretin daily for 12 weeks, while patients treated with narrowband ultraviolet B were offered thrice weekly treatments. Mean adherence to acitretin decreased steadily (slope −0.24 uses/week) from 93.6 % initially to 54.4 % at the end of the 12-week study period. Only 1 (4.5 %) of the 22 participants was 100 % adherent to the regimen. Mean adherence to home phototherapy remained steady with 2–3 treatments per week and only a small decline from 2.4 treatments in the first study week to 2.1 treatments at week 12. In total, 81 % used their phototherapy units at least twice a week, and 44 % used their units at least three times per week [43]. Despite three treatment days a week, dosing was suboptimal and consequently liable to produce suboptimal therapeutic outcomes. Lamps for home treatment should meet the same recognised technical standards as in hospital clinics, which may not always be the case.

Light treatment is an "attack treatment", typically given for a shorter period when psoriasis flares up. The treatment is unrealistic for longer periods or for chronic treatment. Due to excessive demand, treatment clinics cannot offer treatment on a weekly basis, and therefore, it is important that patients adhere to their appointments. Treatment can be inconvenient and costly for the patient; therefore, home phototherapy could, in theory, be an option for patients as an ultimately custom-tailored treatment regimen with improved adherence and, subsequently, a more effective treatment. However, home phototherapy launched decades ago has not passed the test of time and is rarely used.

It is conceivable that phototherapy practised in the routine is a "semi-therapy" of limited and variable efficiency because the full therapeutic potential would require daily doses of light, which cannot be offered. A practice with light treatments scattered over weeks is systematic underdosing of the treatment and a foundation for poor adherence, thus bound to produce inferior therapeutic outcome.

Heliotherapy, balneotherapy and climatotherapy at the Dead Sea bordering Israel and Jordan are an integrated and intensified form of phototherapy with sun combined with other therapeutic elements. Treatment courses at the Dead Sea, which is located 300 m under Mediterranean Sea level, have been practised for thousands of years. Treatments include sun filtered by the special atmosphere of the Dead Sea, bathing in water saturated with salt, mental relaxation and patient education. Psoriasis patients are offered 4 weeks treatment courses closely supervised by dermatology nurses and dermatologists. Treatment is disciplined with six fixed treatment days a week and a voluntary treatment on day 7. Under this setting, it is ensured that adherence to treatment is optimised and high. The sun is, along with mental relaxation, considered the critical elements of the treatment, and salts a supportive treatment helping descaling. A report by the Danish Society of Dermatology reviewed the literature on therapeutic outcome of climatherapy and found the treatment very efficient, matching the efficacy of biologics with fast or faster onset of action. Reoccurrence and variable activity after a few months may be expected for a time-limited "attack" treatment of a chronic disease. A total of 442 enrolled patients achieved a major improvement in their PASI score [44]. This treatment needs follow-up monitoring and treatment if or when relapse occurs. However, relapse has been documented to be milder than after hospitalisation with intensive treatment [44].

Climatotherapy is, from the adherence perspective, a special therapeutic approach and can be considered an "adherence school", primarily based on sun but nevertheless with patient education in disciplined treatment as an equally important treatment goal. The remarkably high effectiveness of the treatment documents the effect of optimised treatment discipline and also illustrates the high power of phototherapy in alleviating psoriasis when light is administered 6 or 7 days a week contrasting the diluted and weak regimen used in today's routine of light therapy in hospital clinics.

10.6   Adherence in Hospitalised Patients and in Patients Under Strict Control

Medication errors may occur during hospitalisation, however, as exceptional events. According to clinicians' experiences, patients treated by professionals in hospital stationary units have an improved adherence rate compared to patient treatment performed under outpatient conditions. Certain treatments, for instance, tar treatment that is still used in recalcitrant cases of psoriasis, can for practical reasons only be given in hospital/clinic settings. The hospital setting allows complicated treatment schedules with combinations of different treatments and adjustments guided by response and side effects. However, under outpatient conditions, only very motivated and qualified patients can follow these complicated schedules. Thus, from the adherence point of view, institutionalised treatment with strict control is a fulfilment of perfection, a fact that is not attainable under the economic constraints of today.

In the field of dermatology, there has been a constant move away from hospital-based treatments to outpatient and private clinic-based treatments. Equally, a number of new and highly efficient medications such as methotrexate and biologics have been introduced. However, despite the theoretical potential of these treatments, treatments taken in the home may result in unsatisfactory adherence resulting in substandard treatment. Light therapy is a quite cumbersome treatment and an example illustrating that treatment provided at outpatient facilities easily can become underdosed because it is undermined by patient's interest in comfort, opting for fewer visits and thereby depreciating treatment and dose. The high efficacy of climatotherapy, as administered in the region of the Dead Sea, under strict control of dermatology staff and under conditions which mimic hospitalisation, illustrates the effect of disciplinary treatment at its best. The ranking of psoriasis patients' adherence and treatment modalities is illustrated in Fig. 10.2.

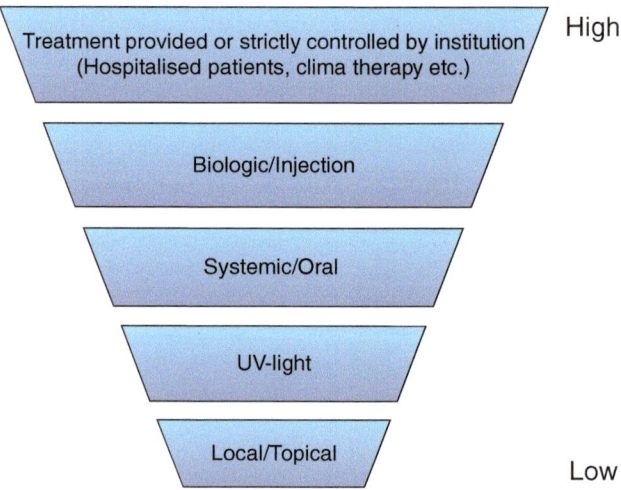

Fig. 10.2 Psoriasis, ranking of adherence and treatment modalities

10.7 Physician-Patient Interaction and Instruments to Improve Adherence to Treatment of Psoriasis

Instruments to improve adherence to treatment may be selective and dependent on the precise treatment. Treatments should be shaped to suit the individual's life and personality. Previous paragraphs have addressed treatment-specific instruments, and the following paragraph will outline general instruments to improve adherence which doctors can take inspiration from and implement to suit the individual patient.

10.7.1 Relationship Between Physician and Patient

The relationship is of utmost importance. Confidence and satisfaction with the scheduled therapy can lead to improved adherence, which again can lead to greater improvement of psoriasis and quality of life [45].

Four hundred ninety-five patients with psoriasis changed to a different dermatologist with a mean of 4.2 times. The most frequent reasons for psoriasis patients changing their dermatologists were lack of efficacy of the prescribed topical treatment (43%) and lack of confidence in the physician (15%) [4].

Physicians' knowledge of psoriasis and persuasiveness will, in all possibility, enhance the quality of treatment. In a questionnaire-based study, 1884 psoriasis patients reported their experiences with psoriasis and their relationship with the doctor [3]. The majority of patients (81%) said they had received clear instructions from their doctors; however, approximately a third sensed their doctor did not take their psoriasis seriously. Also, approximately one third reported lack of help with their psoriasis problem. A comparison of patients' ratings of dermatologists and general practitioners showed dermatologists to be rated slightly more positively. The same authors studied 56 psoriasis patients and reported that 71% consulted a dermatologist more often, 13% a general practitioner (GP), 4% a combination of different medical professionals, 2% a rheumatologist and 11% not regularly seeing any doctor at the present time [3].

Early follow-up consultations are important to encourage patients' treatment behaviour in the direction of better adherence. This is described as the *Hawthorne effect* (the observer effect) where individuals modify or improve an aspect of their behaviour in response to their awareness of being observed [46]. Patients' adherence to treatment decreases between visits and increases before consultations [47–49]. A study from the USA showed quite serious underuse of early follow-up visits of psoriasis patients [50]. Mean length of time to first follow-up visit was 153 days for adults and 142 days for children, which, obviously, is inadequate for any treatment of psoriasis. This is a missed opportunity to improve patient adherence to treatment and treatment outcome, which depends on the ever-changing state of disease accompanied by adjustments of the treatment [50]. Contact by email or phone may be beneficial for the patient-physician relationship and the monitoring of disease and treatment and improve adherence in cases where early follow-up visits cannot be practised. A dermatology nurse could be granted an active role in treatment monitoring aiming at an ever-optimal treatment by the patient in the home. A 12-week study period from Italy of 20 patients with psoriasis on the effects of daily text messages with reminders and educational tools showed significantly improvement to adherence to treatment and to reduction of disease severity, followed by improved quality of life in the active group compared with a control group not granted this service [51].

Doctors are the technical specialists in psoriasis and psoriasis treatment and the patients are the specialists in each individual case including factors related to lifestyle and personal priorities. Much depends on *overcoming the information gap from physician to patient and from patient to physician.* It has been demonstrated that conveyance of basic information concerning diagnosis and medical treatment often is not efficient. Post-consultation investigations among patients after visits to dermatologists revealed that 64 % were familiar with their diagnosis, 55 % were knowledgeable of the scheduled duration of treatment, 71 % were familiar with the number of daily topical applications and 67 % were aware of the detailed dosing of applications [52]. Patients could only recall one third of de facto given information after consultations. These results illustrate the need for more precise, simpler and more understandable patient information provided by the doctor to the patient during a consultation. Patients' precise knowledge of their diagnosis, symptoms, expected spontaneous development of disease and expected effect of active treatment and the side effects are essential in providing any treatment of psoriasis and a matter of good performance of the doctor. A high level of perceived information helps improve adherence to treatment.

There are many factors involved concerning psoriasis patients' low adherence levels (Fig. 10.3). To improve adherence and thus clinical outcomes, solutions must be multifaceted [53].

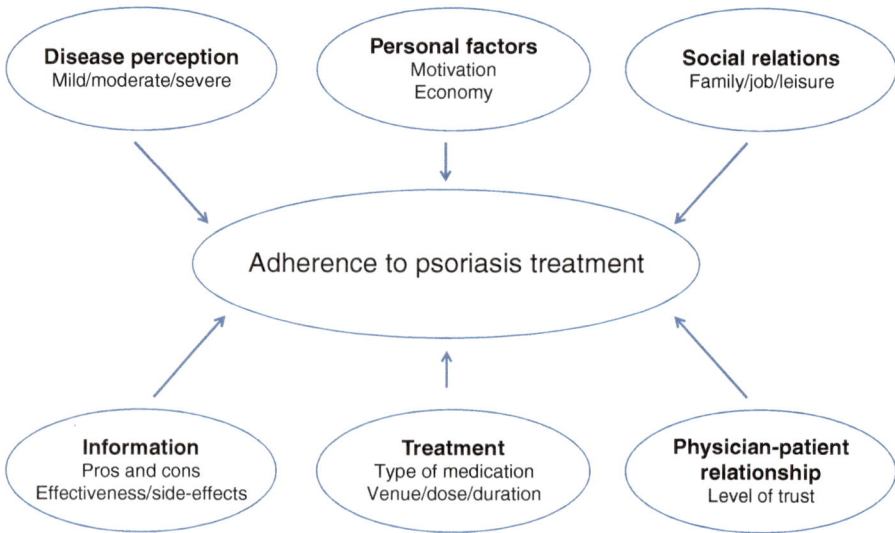

Fig. 10.3 General factors influencing psoriasis patients' adherence to treatment

10.8 Conclusion

Patients with psoriasis, independent of country and health system, are among the typically less adherent segment of dermatology patients. A number of instruments to improve adherence to treatment of psoriasis are available and directly applicable to routine therapy. Some instruments are selected and dependent on the specific type of treatment (Fig. 10.2) and primarily the responsibility of the doctor; others rely on general principles with a need to become materialised and individualised and shaped to the patient and the precise situation and therefore dependent on the active participation of the patient and the provider of treatment (Fig. 10.3). Perfection of treatment in each individual case depends on awareness, insight and mutual understanding, and of both doctor and patient working together in a balanced and qualified interaction where both parties contribute.

References

1. Zachariae R, Claus O, Zachariae C, Lei U, Pedersen AF (2008) Affective and sensory dimensions of pruritus severity: associations with psychological symptoms and quality of life in psoriasis patients. Acta Derm Venereol 88:121–127
2. Dubertret L, Mrowietz U, Ranki A, van de Kerkhof PC, Chimenti S, Lotti T, Schäfer G, EUROPSO Patient Survey Group (2006) European patient perspectives on the impact of psoriasis: the EUROPSO patient membership survey. Br J Dermatol 155:729–736
3. Bewley A, Burrage DM, Ersser SJ, Hansen M, Ward C (2014) Identifying individual psychosocial and adherence support needs in patients with psoriasis: a multinational two-stage qualitative and quantitative study. J Eur Acad Dermatol Venereol 28:763–770
4. Burroni AG, Fassino M, Torti A, Visentin E (2015) How do disease perception, treatment features, and dermatologist-patient relationship impact on patients assuming topical treatment? An Italian survey. Patient Relat Outcome Meas 16:9–17
5. Feldman SR (2013) Disease burden and treatment adherence in psoriasis patients. Cutis 92:258–263
6. Eastman WJ, Malahias S, Delconte J, DiBenedetti D (2014) Assessing attributes of topical vehicles for the treatment of acne, atopic dermatitis, and plaque psoriasis. Cutis 94:46–53
7. Puig L, Carrascosa JM, Belinchón I, Fernández-Redondo V, Carretero G, Ruiz-Carrascosa JC, Careaga JM, de la Cueva P, Gárate MT, Ribera M, Panel de Expertos del Consenso Delphi sobre Tratamiento tópico de la psoriasis, Grupo de Psoriasis de la Academia Española de Dermatología y Venereología (2013) Adherence and patient satisfaction with topical treatment in psoriasis, and the use, and organoleptic properties of such treatments: a Delphi study with an expert panel and members of the psoriasis group of the Spanish Academy of dermatology and venereology. Actas Dermosifiliogr 104:488–496
8. Storm A, Andersen SE, Benfeldt E, Serup J (2008) One in 3 prescriptions are never redeemed: primary nonadherence in an outpatient clinic. J Am Acad Dermatol 59:27–33
9. Storm A, Benfeldt E, Andersen SE, Serup J (2008) A prospective study of patient adherence to topical treatments: 95% of patients underdose. J Am Acad Dermatol 59:975–980
10. Brown KK, Rehmus WE, Kimball AB (2006) Determining the relative importance of patient motivations for nonadherence to topical corticosteroid therapy in psoriasis. J Am Acad Dermatol 55:607–613
11. Devaux S, Castela A, Archier E, Gallini A, Joly P, Misery L, Aractingi S, Aubin F, Bachelez H, Cribier B, Jullien D, Le Maître M, Richard MA, Ortonne JP, Paul C (2012) Adherence to topical treatment in psoriasis: a systematic literature review. J Eur Acad Dermatol Venereol 26:61–67

12. Ulff E, Maroti M, Kettis-Lindblad A, Kjellgren KI, Ahlner J, Ring L, Serup J (2007) Single application of a fluorescent test cream by healthy volunteers: assessment of treated and neglected body sites. Br J Dermatol 156:974–978
13. Schaefer H, Redelmeier TE (1996) Skin barrier: principles of percutaneous absorption. Basel, Karger
14. Bronaugh RL, Maibach HI (2005) Percutaneous absorption, drugs-cosmetics-mechanisms-methodology, vol 55, 4th edn. Taylor and Francis Group, Boca Raton
15. Ulff E, Maroti M, Serup J (2013) Fluorescent cream used as an educational intervention to improve the effectiveness of self-application by patients with atopic dermatitis. J Dermatolog Treat 24:268–271
16. Gartner L, Tarras-Wahlberg C (1984) A double-blind controlled evaluation of diproderm cream 0.05%, twice a day treatment in comparison with once a day treatment in eczema. J Int Med Res 12:59–61
17. Fouéré S, Adjadj L, Pawin H (2005) How patients experience psoriasis: results from a European survey. J Eur Acad Dermatol Venereol 19:2–6
18. Halioua B, Maury Le Breton A, de Fontaubert A, Roussel ME, Stalder JF (2015) Treatment refusal among patients with psoriasis. J Dermatolog Treat 26:396–400
19. Finch T, Shim TN, Roberts L, Johnson O (2015) Treatment satisfaction among patients with moderate-to-severe psoriasis. J Clin Aesthet Dermatol 8:26–30
20. Schaarschmidt ML, Kromer C, Herr R, Schmieder A, Goerdt S, Peitsch WK (2015) Treatment satisfaction of patients with psoriasis. Acta Derm Venereol 95:572–578
21. Saeki H, Imafuku S, Abe M, Shintani Y, Onozuka D, Hagihara A, Katoh N, Murota H, Takeuchi S, Sugaya M, Tanioka M, Kaneko S, Masuda K, Hiragun T, Inomata N, Kitami Y, Tsunemi Y, Abe S, Kobayashi M, Morisky DE, Furue M (2015) Poor adherence to medication as assessed by the Morisky medication adherence scale-8 and low satisfaction with treatment in 237 psoriasis patients. J Dermatol 42:367–372
22. Roenigk HH (1994) Methotrexate. In: Dubertret L. Psoriasis (ed.). ISED Italy. pp 162–173
23. Inzinger M, Weger W, Heschl B, Salmhofer W, Quehenberger F, Wolf P (2013) Methotrexate vs. fumaric acid esters in moderate-to-severe chronic plaque psoriasis: data registry report on the efficacy under daily life conditions. J Eur Acad Dermatol Venereol 27:861–866
24. Zachariae C, Mørk NJ, Reunala T, Lorentzen H, Falk E, Karvonen SL, Johannesson A, Claréus B, Skov L, Mørk G, Walker S, Qvitzau S (2008) The combination of etanercept and methotrexate increases the effectiveness of treatment in active psoriasis despite inadequate effect of methotrexate therapy. Acta Derm Venereol 88:495–501
25. Migliore A, Cusano F, Bianchi G, Malara G, Epis O, De Pità O (2015) Management of psoriatic arthritis: should the interaction between dermatologists and rheumatologists in clinical practice be intensified? J Biol Regul Homeost Agents 29:547–561
26. Nikiphorou E, Negoescu A, Fitzpatrick JD, Goudie CT, Badcock A, Östör AJ, Malaviya AP (2014) Indispensable or intolerable? Methotrexate in patients with rheumatoid and psoriatic arthritis: a retrospective review of discontinuation rates from a large UK cohort. Clin Rheumatol 33:609–614
27. McHugh NJ (2015) Early psoriatic arthritis. Rheum Dis Clin North Am 41:615–622
28. You HS, Kim GW, Cho HH, Kim WJ, Mun JH, Song M, Kim HS, Ko HC, Kim MB, Lee SG, Lee IS, Kim BS (2015) Screening for psoriatic arthritis in Korean psoriasis patients using the psoriatic arthritis screening evaluation questionnaire. Ann Dermatol 27:265–268
29. Roll A, Reich K, Boer A (2007) Use of fumaric acid esters in psoriasis. Indian J Dermatol Venereol Leprol 73:133–137
30. Ismail N, Collins P, Rogers S, Kirby B, Lally A (2014) Drug survival of fumaric acid esters for psoriasis: a retrospective study. Br J Dermatol 171:397–402
31. Swimberghe S, Ghislain PD, Daci E, Allewaert K, Denhaerynck K, Hermans C, Pacheco C, Vancayzeele S, MacDonald K, Abraham I (2013) Clinical, quality of life, patient adherence, and safety outcomes of short-course (12 weeks) treatment with cyclosporine in patients with severe psoriasis (the practice study). Ann Dermatol 25:28–35
32. Nast A, Gisondi P, Ormerod AD, Saiag P, Smith C, Spuls PI, Arenberger P, Bachelez H, Barker J, Dauden E, de Jong EM, Feist E, Jacobs A, Jobling R, Kemény L, Maccarone M, Mrowietz U,

Papp KA, Paul C, Reich K, Rosumeck S, Talme T, Thio HB, van de Kerkhof P, Werner RN, Yawalkar N (2015) European S3-guidelines on the systemic treatment of psoriasis vulgaris – update 2015 – short version – EDF in cooperation with EADV and IPC. J Eur Acad Dermatol Venereol 29:2277–2294

33. Poulin Y, Papp KA, Wasel NR et al (2010) A Canadian online survey to evaluate awareness and treatment satisfaction in individuals with moderate to severe plaque psoriasis. Int J Dermatol 49:1368–1375

34. DiBonaventura M, Wagner S, Waters H, Carter C (2010) Treatment patterns and perceptions of treatment attributes, satisfaction and effectiveness among patients with psoriasis. J Drugs Dermatol 9:938–944

35. Jones-Caballero M, Unaeze J, Penas PF, Stern RS (2007) Use of biological agents in patients with moderate to severe psoriasis: a cohort based perspective. Arch Dermatol 143:846–850

36. Mahler R, Jackson C, Ijacu H (2009) The burden of psoriasis and barriers to satisfactory care: results from a Canadian patient survey. J Cutan Med Surg 13:283–293

37. Bhosle MJ, Feldman SR, Camacho FT, Whitmire TJ, Nahata MC, Balkrishnan R (2006) Medication adherence and health care costs associated with biologics in Medicaid- enrolled patients with psoriasis. J Dermatolog Treat 17:294–301

38. Gisondi P, Tessari G, Di Mercurio M et al (2013) Retention rate of systemic drugs in patients with chronic plaque psoriasis. Clin Dermatol 1:8–14

39. Ross C, Marshman G, Grillo M, Stanford T (2015) Biological therapies for psoriasis: adherence and outcome analysis from a clinical perspective. Australas J Dermatol (Epub ahead of print)

40. Drugs.com (visited 3 Dec 2015), searched titles: Ustekinumab, infliximab, adalimumab and etanercept

41. Zhang M, Brenneman SK, Carter CT, Essoi BL, Farahi K, Johnson MP, Lee S, Olson WH (2015) Patient-reported treatment satisfaction and choice of dosing frequency with biologic treatment for moderate to severe plaque psoriasis. Patient Prefer Adherence 16(8):777–784

42. Kalia S, Toosi B, Bansback N et al (2014) Assessing adherence with phototherapy protocols. J Am Acad Dermatol 71:1259–1261

43. Yentzer BA, Yelverton CB, Pearce DJ et al (2008) Adherence to acitretin and home narrow-band ultraviolet B phototherapy in patients with psoriasis. J Am Acad Dermatol 59:577–581

44. Lings C, Kragballe K (2008) Klimabehandling til psoriasis (Eng: climatherapy for psoriasis), Århus Hospital, Denmark

45. Carroll CL, Feldman SR, Camacho FT, Balkrishnan R (2004) Better medication adherence results in greater improvement in severity of psoriasis. Br J Dermatol 151:895–897

46. Davis SA, Feldman SR (2013) Using Hawthorne effects to improve adherence in clinical practice: lessons from clinical trials. JAMA Dermatol 149:490–491

47. Gelfand JM, Wang S, Takeshita J, Robertson AD et al (2013) Response to "Using Effects to Improve Adherence in Clinical Practice: Lessons from Clinical Trials". JAMA Dermatol 149:490–491

48. Cramer JA, Scheyer RD, Mattson RH (1990) Compliance declines between clinic visits. Arch Intern Med 150:1509–1510

49. Feldman SR, Camacho FT, Krejci-Manwaring J, Carroll CL, Balkrishnan R (2007) Adherence to topical therapy increases around the time of office visits. J Am Acad Dermatol 57:81–83

50. Davis SA, Lin HC, Yu CH, Balkrishnan R, Feldman SR (2014) Underuse of early follow-up visits: a missed opportunity to improve patients' adherence. J Drugs Dermatol 13:833–836

51. Balato N, Megna M, Di Costanzo L, Balato A, Ayala F (2013) Educational and motivational support service: a pilot study for mobile-phone-based interventions in patients with psoriasis. Br J Dermatol 168:201–205

52. Storm A, Benfeldt E, Andersen SE, Serup J (2009) Basic drug information given by physicians is deficient, and patients' knowledge low. J Dermatolog Treat 20:190–193

53. Zschocke I, Mrowietz U, Karakasili E, Reich K (2014) Non-adherence and measures to improve adherence in the topical treatment of psoriasis. J Eur Acad Dermatol Venereol 28:4–9

Chapter 11
Adherence in Atopic Dermatitis

Hélène Aubert and Sébastien Barbarot

11.1 Introduction

As defined by the UK Working Party's diagnostic criteria [1], atopic dermatitis (AD), also known as atopic eczema, is a relapsing, chronic, inflammatory, cutaneous disorder that occurs mainly in childhood and sometimes persists into adulthood [2]. AD currently affects 10–30 % of children worldwide [3, 4]. It is a public health concern because of its prevalence, cost, and impact on quality of life. Atopic eczema in children can indeed have a profound effect on quality of life, causing major sleep disruption for the child and family and interfering with normal development, education, and play. Thus, the broad impact of AD warrants optimization of relevant support services.

Topical corticosteroids remain the mainstay of treatment regimen in atopic dermatitis because of their ability to reduce inflammation and erythema. They are often required for months or years to control the disease and prevent recurring flares. During asymptomatic disease periods, topical emollient use is also critical to prevent relapse.

Adherence to treatment in this chronic condition is the cornerstone of successful treatment.

Adherence to treatment is classically defined as "the process by which patients take their medication as prescribed," and nonadherence to medications is defined as "late or non-initiation of the prescribed treatment, sub-optimal implementation of the dosing regimen or early discontinuation of the treatment" [5].

However, adherence to treatment is a tricky concept to define in AD.

H. Aubert, MD • S. Barbarot, MD, PhD (✉)
Dermatology Department, Ecole de l'atopie, CHU de Nantes, CHU Hôtel Dieu,
Nantes 44035, France
e-mail: sebastien.barbarot@chu-nantes.fr

© Springer International Publishing Switzerland 2016
S.A. Davis (ed.), *Adherence in Dermatology*,
DOI 10.1007/978-3-319-30994-1_11

122

H. Aubert and S. Barbarot

11.1.1 Adherence to Treatment Is a Moving Target in AD

Indeed, one of the key points of the therapeutic strategy in AD is the fact that the quantity and frequency of topical treatment to be applied vary with the intensity of the disease over time. The patient has to adapt his treatment to his daily skin condition. Consequently, adherence should be evaluated in conjunction with these fluctuations of intensity. For instance, if the patient is free from inflammatory skin lesions on a given day, it is normal for that patient not to use topical steroid: this should not be considered as poor adherence. Therefore, a practitioner may have prescribed a certain amount of topical steroid for daily application and realized at the follow-up visit that the patient has only applied half of the prescribed amount. It does not mean necessarily that the patient was not adherent; it may simply mean that he did not need to use the treatment because his disease severity was low between the two visits.

11.1.2 Adherence to Treatment Is Complex to Assess in AD

It is actually difficult to assess a patient with AD as "adherent" or "nonadherent." Indeed, the goals of patients and doctors are often different in AD. While doctors often seek to achieve an objective improvement of severity scores, patients use discomfort thresholds beyond which they decide to start treatment application. These thresholds are variable from one patient to another.

Adherence in dermatology is a complex problem. It seems difficult to define it within the specific field of AD and even harder to evaluate or monitor it.

Moreover, adherence in AD is technically difficult to evaluate as in other chronic skin diseases. Pharmacy refill rates and weighing medications are objective measures; so is the electronic medication monitoring device (MEMS cap), but yet medication consumption is assumed but not confirmed [5, 6]. The patient self-report methods often used to assess adherence are more subjective.

Due to the inherent subjectivity of the patient, constant adaptations to the fluctuating severity of the disease, and lack of appropriate technical devices, the perfect way to assess adherence in AD does not yet exist.

11.2 What Do We Know About Adherence in AD?

Topical corticosteroids remain the mainstay of treatment in AD. AD requires treatment over an extended period of time. Topical corticosteroids are highly effective treatment, but the effectiveness of treatment is limited by poor adherence as in other chronic conditions. Poor adherence seems to be the major cause of treatment failure in AD. There has been little work assessing adherence to complex treatment regimens in AD which often involve emollient products (cream/ointment, bath oil, and soap), two or more topical steroids (e.g., face, hair, and body), and dressings.

In clinical trials assessing efficacy or tolerance of topical treatments in AD, adherence to medication is rarely an outcome and is often presumed to be good. It is the same for systemic treatments in AD about which data on adherence are very rare. It is known that clinical trials can improve adherence by several methods, such as reimbursement and multiple study visits.

11.2.1 In the Literature, Some Data Are Available on Adherence to Topical Treatment in AD in Clinical Trials Setting

Krejci-Manwaring et al. performed in 2007 a study to specifically measure adherence in AD children [7]. In this study, 37 children were given 0.1 % triamcinolone ointment twice daily for 8 weeks. The adherence was electronically monitored (MEMS cap) and patients were not informed of the adherence monitoring. Mean adherence from the baseline to the end of the study was only 32 %.

Another study in 2010 by Yentzer et al. on 41 patients with mild to moderate AD found that mean adherence to twice daily application of desonide hydrogel decreased from 81 % on day 1 to 50 % on day 27 [8]. Adherence was assessed by electronic devices in this study and it is important to mention that subjects received a phone call on day 3.

A large study by Furue et al. of about 3,096 patients with cutaneous diseases studied adherence using the Morisky Medication Adherence Scale 8 (MMAS-8). One thousand three hundred twenty-seven patients had AD, and 76.9 % of the patients with AD had MMAS-8 score under 6 (defined by the authors as low adherence). Only 5.9 % of the patients with AD were highly adherent to topical treatments [9].

Two studies were designed to determine whether a short course of treatment with high-potency corticosteroid would improve adherence compared to longer treatment.

In the first study by Hix et al. [10], ten patients with mild to moderate AD were instructed to apply fluocinonide cream 0.1 % twice daily for 5 days. Adherence was self-reported and electronically monitored. The median adherence rate in this study from the electronic monitors was 40 %. In the second study by Yentzer [11], 20 participants with mild to severe AD were instructed to use fluocinonide cream 0.1 % twice daily for three consecutive days for a total of six doses. Disease severity was assessed at baseline, day 3, day 7, and day 14. Electronic monitoring was used to measure adherence to treatment. Median adherence to treatment over the 3-day period was 100 %.

Regarding maintenance treatment in AD, Torrelo et al. [12] performed in Spain in 2009–2010 a national, multicenter, cross-sectional, epidemiological study in adults and children with moderate or severe AD of at least 16 months' duration who were receiving maintenance therapy. This topical treatment was prescribed according to the dermatologist's criteria, following the routine clinical practice of each hospital. The Morisky Medication Adherence Scale was used to assess adherence. The authors studied 141 children and 141 adults. While treatment satisfaction was high in both groups, adherence was poor (18.4–42.6 % in children and 14.9–27.0 % in adults).

Ortiz de frutos et al. performed a study to evaluate adherence among AD patients in Spain [13]. This was a multicenter, cross-sectional, epidemiological study with the participation of adults (age >16 years; $n = 125$) and children (age, 2–15 years, $n = 116$). Patients had a history of at least 12 months of moderate to severe AD. The patients indicated how often they followed medical recommendations for AD control on a 6-point Likert-type scale ranging from 1 (always) to 6 (rarely or never). Although patients stated that they followed medical recommendations (always, 35.2 %; nearly always, 40 %), a significant percentage of patients did not apply recommended treatments correctly: in 47.2 % of adults and 39.7 % of children, pharmacological therapy was not initiated at flare onset, and an additional 13.6 % of adults and 17.2 % of children had not applied any topical pharmacotherapy despite the presence of a moderate to severe flare.

As well as in other chronic dermatological diseases, adherence in AD appears to be poor, especially in maintenance treatment which is essential to reach long-term control of the disease.

11.3   Factors Influencing Adherence in AD

11.3.1   Factors Associated to Adherence to Treatments in Chronic Diseases

A wide range of factors have been associated with poor adherence in AD.

Several dimensions are shared with other chronic diseases: socioeconomic factors (poverty, insecurity, illiteracy, poor education, unemployment, isolation), factors related to the health system, factors associated with the disease (disease severity and symptoms, prognosis, and comorbidities), treatment-related factors (complexity, duration, side effects experienced or feared, previous treatment failures), and patient-related factors.

The patient-related factors that are associated with poor adherence are forgetfulness, low motivation, low sense of self-efficacy, poor knowledge of treatment, poor understanding or acceptance of the disease, and anxiety related to the fear of side effects or addiction [14, 15].

11.3.2   Factors Associated to Adherence to Topical Treatment in Chronic Skin Diseases

Some factors are due to topical medication and common with other dermatological diseases (psoriasis, acne). As most topical therapies are used for the management of highly symptomatic disease, it may be assumed that adherence to topical treatment is higher for topical treatment versus oral treatments. As we have seen above, that is not the case.

Patient-related factors associated with poor adherence to topical treatment are younger age, concerned about safety and psychiatric comorbidities, frequency of hospital visits, experience of drug effectiveness, and overall satisfaction with treatment [9]. Medication-related factors are side effects and higher frequency of administration, misbeliefs or misunderstanding about the disease and treatment regimen, complexity of the treatment regimen, the fact that it is time-consuming to apply topical medications, and the nonaesthetic and galenic nature of the topical treatment [5, 16].

11.3.3 Factors Associated with Adherence to Treatments in AD

Some factors that impact adherence are specific to AD. Indeed, the patient has to adapt his treatment to his skin condition every day. That is why the patients need to acquire abilities about the treatment: which lesions are eczema or dry skin, which topical treatment to use and how to use it, and when to start the treatment and when to stop. For Beattie et al. [17], the main factor of poor adherence in AD is the lack of knowledge about treatment management.

The involvement of the family plays a crucial role in the treatment of children with AD. Parents are frequently the primary caregivers. The chronic management of a disease that requires long-lasting caregiver efforts may build up caregiver burden. In a qualitative study in mothers of children with AD, it appears that convenience of medication use and caregiver education are key domains affecting treatment adherence [18].

Patient- or parent-doctor relationship is another crucial domain affecting adherence in AD identified by several authors [18, 19]. Another factor of poor adherence may be the child refusal of therapy or child resistance [20].

Last but not least, the high cost of the creams and above all emollients can be an obstacle to their use.

As AD is a frequent skin disease, patients have many health beliefs about the disease and also about the treatment. Fear of topical corticosteroid side effects is very frequent in clinical practice in the field of AD.

11.4 Topical Corticosteroid (TCS) Phobia

11.4.1 TCS Phobia Definition

Corticosteroid phobia is the dedicated term to describe all types of fear related to steroid use. This notion of fear or reluctance to the use of corticosteroids is called in the literature "corticophobia." It is not really a phobia in the psychiatric sense because that fear is sometimes reasoned.

11.4.2   TCS Phobia Frequency

The term "corticophobia" was used for the first time in 1979 by L. Tuft [21] about fears of doctors against inhaled steroids in asthma and the potentially negative impact of these fears on the management of patients. Some authors further expanded this notion to topical steroids [22, 23].

In routine clinical practice, it is not unusual for patients to express fear or anxiety about using TCS and TCS phobia appears to be common.

Fischer in 1996 found that 40 % of patients thought TCS were dangerous [24]. In a questionnaire study involving 200 patients with AD [25], Charman et al. found that 73 % of the patients or parents of children with AD reported being worried about using TCS. In 2006, using the same questionnaire, Hon et al. [26] found that 60 % of 233 patients had fears about TCS. In Japan, 38.3 % of the caregivers were reluctant to use TCS on their children's skin [27].

In a recent study in France, the prevalence of corticophobia was even more important, since eight out of ten patients reported fears about the use of topical corticosteroids in AD [28].

Notably, TCS phobia rates differed in China [26], the UK [25], Japan [27], and France, highlighting cultural differences in how the general population perceives corticosteroids.

TCS phobia was further studied in AD and seems less common in psoriasis. However, in Brown's study, fear of side effects of TCS is associated with poor adherence in patients with psoriasis [29].

11.4.3   TCS Phobia Features

The intensity of TCS phobia varies from one patient to another. Although the majority of patients had moderate fear, some had extreme anxieties. Patients mainly fear the side effects of corticosteroids. Some patients had specific fears about TCS use, most of which concerned adverse events, predominantly cutaneous side effects. Some patients worried about systemic side effects, principally growth retardation and weight gain. Some of these dreaded side effects do exist (skin atrophy, depigmentation, superinfection), but they are overestimated and overinterpreted by patients [30, 31].

Corticophobia is also related to patients' worries about how to apply TCS (how much, how long, and where). These fears of doing the wrong thing are related to the fear of the occurrence of a side effect and have their genesis in the quality of the information. A major fear of patients concerns the risk of dependency (inability to stop treatment) or addiction (higher doses to achieve the same effect). The risk of developing a dependency or addiction is related to the feeling of loss of efficacy of treatment often reported by patients.

However, some patients have nonspecific concerns. Many patients said they did not know the side effects of TCS but were still afraid of using them. According to

Charman et al. [25], 24 % of their patients worried about long-term nonspecific adverse events. In the study of Aubert-Wastiaux et al., 47.8 % of the patients have indeterminate worries [28]. These nonspecific fears might be associated with a lack of information, with information discrepancies, or with the term "steroid." Notably, some patients who did not admit to being worried about using TCS expressed TCS phobia through their behaviors. Indeed, many patients reported waiting until their AD got worse or applying TCS only as a last resort to avoid potential side effects. Thus, TCS phobia is a complex phenomenon that manifests as specific or indeterminate fears or only as specific behaviors.

11.4.4 Origins of TCS Phobia

First, verbal information given by providers seems to play an important role. Indeed, a lack of clear advice was significantly correlated with TCS phobia. Inconsistent information about the quantity to use, the area to treat, and treatment duration induces worries. Patients reported discrepancies concerning all these treatment aspects among dermatologists, between dermatologists and general practitioners, and between practitioners and pharmacists [28]. These variations might be attributable to advances in our understanding of TCS and their safety over the years and perhaps even reflect TCS phobia among providers themselves, especially those trained a long time ago.

11.4.5 Characteristics of Patients with Corticophobia

TCS phobia is not associated with either the characteristics of AD (duration, impact, and severity) or the patient (age, sex, or type of consultation). Thus, TCS phobia can affect all patients with AD [27, 28].

11.4.6 Impact of TCS Phobia on Adherence

Several studies confirm the impact of TCS phobia on treatment adherence: the greater the fear, the poorer the compliance.

Several authors [17, 24, 25] attributed many therapeutic failures to poor adherence and suggested that TCS phobia played a contributory role. Only Ohya et al. [19] failed to detect an impact on adherence.

TCS phobia and treatment adherence are associated concepts but remain separate: patients can be adherent to treatment and still have worries about it. A patient may have fears or worries about TCS and still be adherent: this is a source of anxiety and poor treatment experiences. The link between corticophobia and adherence is essential and supports the need for a systematic exploration of corticophobia among AD patients. However, patients recognize the benefits of treatment despite their fears. The benefit/risk balance of treatment should be clearly discussed with the patient.

11.5 How to Improve Adherence in AD

Improving adherence in AD is a crucial point and adherence to topical treatment should always be checked before considering systemic treatments.

Some techniques to improve adherence are shared with other chronic conditions, such as simplifying the treatment regimen or using reminders. Some are common with other dermatological diseases like scheduling early follow-up visits. Indeed, it appears in many studies that adherence to topical therapy increases around the time of office visits [32–35].

The properties of vehicle formulations may influence drug delivery, efficacy, and tolerance profiles of topical medications. Patient preferences vary and the importance of certain aesthetic attributes depends on the disease state, the site of application, and the length and extent of treatment [36]. Following patient preferences may improve patients' willingness to apply therapy as directed and therefore may affect the outcome of treatment. AD patients often report itching and redness with emollient or TCS use [37]. Then, the choice of the vehicle in AD should be made according to patient preferences.

Therapeutic patient education is already used in many chronic diseases. Therapeutic patient education (TPE) is aimed at improving the therapeutic adherence of patients and their families. According to the World Health Organization (WHO) definition, TPE helps patients with chronic disease to acquire or maintain the skills they need to manage their life in the best possible way. In AD, TPE is particularly relevant and should be integrated into the care process to improve patient adherence and quality of life. Topical treatment regimens are often complex, and patients and their families are directly responsible for applying and adapting them to the daily condition of the disease. Therefore, patients need to acquire the skills necessary to self-assess and adapt local treatments for the long-term control of the disease [38].

Patients or parents should acquire knowledge of the disease (disease mechanisms, treatment mechanisms, aggravating factors), practical skills (applying treatment and adapting it to disease severity, self-assessing disease severity), and relational skills (explaining the disease to others, knowing whom to turn to during a flare-up and when to ask for help).

Written action plans, as for asthma, are also very helpful in AD [39].

Demonstration of how to apply topical treatment in AD is also very important. In Cork et al.'s study [40], a specialist dermatology nurse explained and demonstrated how to use all of the topical treatments at the first visit. This education was repeated at subsequent visits depending on the knowledge of the parent. This intervention had a positive impact on adherence and AD severity.

The last specific domain in the way to improve adherence in AD is the management of TCS phobia. As we said above, exploration of TCS phobia among AD should be always done as corticophobia is often not acknowledged spontaneously by patients. It is essential to detect any corticophobia with open questions that are not guilt-inducing (e.g., "I know that patients often have fears about using corticosteroids: what do you think?"). Exploring a patient's perceptions and beliefs about TCS phobia allows information to be targeted individually.

Then the patient should explain his beliefs and causes of fears (previous experience of adverse effects, fear of dependency, loss of efficacy, incoherent speech of providers, lack of explanation on how to use, or vague fears).

Caregivers should give clear and consistent explanations about the disease and treatment (clear detail of how much to apply, where to apply, how long to apply for). The issue of adverse effects must also be assessed. Current advice to patients to apply topical corticosteroid preparations "sparingly" or "thinly" contributes to "steroid phobia," increasing the risk of poor clinical response and treatment failure. Such cautionary advice also overlooks the fact that the vast majority of patients are prescribed topical corticosteroids of mild potency for which the evidence suggests that the risk of harm is minimal [41].

The quality of the patient-doctor relationship is critical to ensuring treatment adherence and patient self-efficacy. Trust in the physician and reassurance about treatment are essential to reduce TCS phobia [28].

11.6 In Conclusion

Adherence in AD is difficult to define and to evaluate. The data available in the literature demonstrate that adherence in AD is low. Lack of knowledge about treatment, patient-doctor relationship, and TCS phobia are the main factors influencing adherence in AD.

References

1. Williams HC, Burney PG, Pembroke AC, Hay RJ (1994) The U.K. working party's diagnostic criteria for atopic dermatitis. III. Independent hospital validation. Br J Dermatol 131(3):406–416
2. Silverberg JI, Hanifin JM (2013) Adult eczema prevalence and associations with asthma and other health and demographic factors: a US population-based study. J Allergy Clin Immunol 132(5):1132–1138
3. Bieber T (2008) Atopic dermatitis. N Engl J Med 358(14):1483–1494, 3 avr
4. Spergel JM (2010) Epidemiology of atopic dermatitis and atopic march in children. Immunol Allergy Clin North Am 30(3):269–280
5. Tan X, Feldman SR, Chang J, Balkrishnan R (2012) Topical drug delivery systems in dermatology: a review of patient adherence issues. Expert Opin Drug Deliv 9(10):1263–1271
6. Koehler AM, Maibach HI (2001) Electronic monitoring in medication adherence measurement. Implications for dermatology. Am J Clin Dermatol 2(1):7–12

7. Krejci-Manwaring J, Tusa MG, Carroll C, Camacho F, Kaur M, Carr D et al (2007) Stealth monitoring of adherence to topical medication: adherence is very poor in children with atopic dermatitis. J Am Acad Dermatol 56(2):211–216

8. Yentzer BA, Camacho FT, Young T, Fountain JM, Clark AR, Feldman SR (2010) Good adherence and early efficacy using desonide hydrogel for atopic dermatitis: results from a program addressing patient compliance. J Drugs Dermatol JDD 9(4):324–329

9. Furue M, Onozuka D, Takeuchi S, Murota H, Sugaya M, Masuda K et al (2015) Poor adherence to oral and topical medication in 3096 dermatological patients as assessed by the Morisky Medication Adherence Scale-8. Br J Dermatol 172(1):272–275

10. Hix E, Gustafson CJ, O'Neill JL, Huang K, Sandoval LF, Harrison J et al (2013) Adherence to a five day treatment course of topical fluocinonide 0.1% cream in atopic dermatitis. Dermatol Online J 19(10):20029

11. Yentzer BA, Ade RA, Fountain JM, Clark AR, Taylor SL, Borgerding E et al (2010) Improvement in treatment adherence with a 3-day course of fluocinonide cream 0.1% for atopic dermatitis. Cutis 86(4):208–213

12. Torrelo A, Ortiz J, Alomar A, Ros S, Pedrosa E, Cuervo J (2013) Health-related quality of life, patient satisfaction, and adherence to treatment in patients with moderate or severe atopic dermatitis on maintenance therapy: the CONDA-SAT study. Actas Dermosifiliogr 104(5):409–417

13. Ortiz de Frutos FJ, Torrelo A, de Lucas R, González MA, Alomar A, Vera Á et al (2014) Patient perspectives on triggers, adherence to medical recommendations, and disease control in atopic dermatitis: the DATOP study. Actas Dermosifiliogr 105(5):487–496

14. Krueger KP, Berger BA, Felkey B (2005) Medication adherence and persistence: a comprehensive review. Adv Ther 22(4):313–356

15. Osterberg L, Blaschke T (2005) Adherence to medication. N Engl J Med 353(5):487–497

16. Gupta G, Mallefet P, Kress DW, Sergeant A (2009) Adherence to topical dermatological therapy: lessons from oral drug treatment. Br J Dermatol 161(2):221–227

17. Beattie PE, Lewis-Jones MS (2003) Parental knowledge of topical therapies in the treatment of childhood atopic dermatitis. Clin Exp Dermatol 28(5):549–553

18. Fenerty SD, O'Neill JL, Gustafson CJ, Feldman SR (2013) Maternal adherence factors in the treatment of pediatric atopic dermatitis. JAMA Dermatol 149(2):229–231

19. Ohya Y, Williams H, Steptoe A, Saito H, Iikura Y, Anderson R et al (2001) Psychosocial factors and adherence to treatment advice in childhood atopic dermatitis. J Invest Dermatol 117(4):852–857

20. Santer M, Burgess H, Yardley L, Ersser SJ, Lewis-Jones S, Muller I et al (2013) Managing childhood eczema: qualitative study exploring carers' experiences of barriers and facilitators to treatment adherence. J Adv Nurs 69(11):2493–2501

21. Tuft L (1979) «Steroid-phobia» in asthma management. Ann Allergy 42(3):152–159

22. David TJ (1987) Steroid scare. Arch Dis Child 62(9):876–878

23. Patterson R, Walker CL, Greenberger PA, Sheridan EP (1989) Prednisonephobia. Allergy Proc Off J Reg State Allergy Soc 10(6):423–428

24. Fischer G (1996) Compliance problems in paediatric atopic eczema. Australas J Dermatol 37(Suppl 1):S10–S13

25. Charman CR, Morris AD, Williams HC (2000) Topical corticosteroid phobia in patients with atopic eczema. Br J Dermatol 142(5):931–936

26. Hon K-LE, Kam W-YC, Leung T-F, Lam M-CA, Wong K-Y, Lee K-CK et al (2006) Steroid fears in children with eczema. Acta Paediatr Oslo Nor 1992 95(11):1451–1455

27. Kojima R, Fujiwara, Matsuda, Narita, Matsubara. Factors associated with steroid pho… [Pediatr Dermatol. 2013 Jan-Feb] – PubMed – NCBI [Internet]. [cité 20 janv 2014]. Disponible sur: http://www.ncbi.nlm.nih.gov/pubmed/22747965

28. Aubert-Wastiaux H, Moret L, Le Rhun A, Fontenoy AM, Nguyen JM, Leux C et al (2011) Topical corticosteroid phobia in atopic dermatitis: a study of its nature, origins and frequency. Br J Dermatol 165(4):808–814

29. Brown KL, Krejci-Manwaring J, Tusa MG, Camacho F, Fleischer AB, Balkrishnan R et al (2008) Poor compliance with topical corticosteroids for atopic dermatitis despite severe disease. Dermatol Online J 14(9):13
30. Thomas KS, Armstrong S, Avery A, Po ALW, O'Neill C, Young S et al (2002) Randomised controlled trial of short bursts of a potent topical corticosteroid versus prolonged use of a mild preparation for children with mild or moderate atopic eczema. BMJ 324(7340):768
31. Van Der Meer JB, Glazenburg EJ, Mulder PG, Eggink HF, Coenraads PJ (1999) The management of moderate to severe atopic dermatitis in adults with topical fluticasone propionate. The Netherlands Adult Atopic Dermatitis Study Group. Br J Dermatol 140(6):1114–1121
32. Davis SA, Lin H-C, Yu C-H, Balkrishnan R, Feldman SR (2014) Underuse of early follow-up visits: a missed opportunity to improve patients' adherence. J Drugs Dermatol JDD 13(7):833–836
33. Shah A, Yentzer BA, Feldman SR (2013) Timing of return office visit affects adherence to topical treatment in patients with atopic dermatitis: an analysis of 5 studies. Cutis 91(2):105–107
34. Carroll CL, Feldman SR, Camacho FT, Manuel JC, Balkrishnan R (2004) Adherence to topical therapy decreases during the course of an 8-week psoriasis clinical trial: commonly used methods of measuring adherence to topical therapy overestimate actual use. J Am Acad Dermatol 51(2):212–216
35. Feldman SR, Camacho FT, Krejci-Manwaring J, Carroll CL, Balkrishnan R (2007) Adherence to topical therapy increases around the time of office visits. J Am Acad Dermatol 57(1):81–83
36. Trookman NS, Rizer RL, Ho ET, Ford RO, Gotz V (2011) The importance of vehicle properties to patients with atopic dermatitis. Cutis 88(1 Suppl):13–17
37. Eastman WJ, Malahias S, Delconte J, DiBenedetti D (2014) Assessing attributes of topical vehicles for the treatment of acne, atopic dermatitis, and plaque psoriasis. Cutis 94(1):46–53
38. Barbarot S, Bernier C, Deleuran M, De Raeve L, Eichenfield L, El Hachem M et al (2013) Therapeutic patient education in children with atopic dermatitis: position paper on objectives and recommendations. Pediatr Dermatol 30(2):199–206
39. Chisolm SS, Taylor SL, Balkrishnan R, Feldman SR (2008) Written action plans: potential for improving outcomes in children with atopic dermatitis. J Am Acad Dermatol 59(4):677–683
40. Cork MJ, Britton J, Butler L, Young S, Murphy R, Keohane SG. Comparison of parent knowledge, therapy utilization and severity of atopic eczema before and after explanation and demonstration of topical therapies by a specialist dermatology nurse. Br J Dermatol 2003;149(3):582–9
41. Bewley A, Dermatology Working Group (2008) Expert consensus: time for a change in the way we advise our patients to use topical corticosteroids. Br J Dermatol 158(5):917–920

Chapter 12
Adherence in Other Dermatologic Conditions

Chantal Jackson and Howard I. Maibach

12.1 Introduction

Adherence is integral to patient health [1]. Moreover, when patients fail to comply with suggested measures, it is economically taxing to the medical community at large [2]. These ideas make it crucial to understand adherence-related behavior. By better understanding compliance, mechanisms geared toward improvement might be established. This chapter discusses adherence in two ways: prevention and treatment. The first manner through which to examine compliance behavior will be in relation to sun-induced skin damage (specifically skin cancer, premature aging, and actinic keratosis), while the second concerns a specific connective tissue disorder, localized scleroderma.

Unique challenges arise in the field of dermatology with regard to patient compliance [2]. For example, myriad forms of media promote a tanned appearance as a representation of youth and vitality, despite the potentially deleterious consequences of achieving such an image [3]. Furthermore, certain types of sun-induced skin damage can take years to develop [4]; thus, the benefit for this desirable appearance might outweigh the negative cost.

Excessive sun exposure is implicated as a primary contributor across a plethora of skin cancer categories [5]. Markedly, proper and adequate sunscreen use has been noted in the prevention of various UV-related skin damage including photoaging, melanoma, and nonmelanoma cancer forms [5]. Despite the knowledge that sunscreen use and other protective measures such as clothing, wearing of hat, and sun avoidance are essential in sun damage deterrence, the incidence of skin cancer is on the rise [6]. Due to this worldwide increase in skin cancer [7], it is highly relevant

Chantal Jackson • H.I. Maibach (✉)
University of California, San Francisco, CA, USA
e-mail: chantaltjackson@gmail.com; MaibachH@derm.ucsf.edu

© Springer International Publishing Switzerland 2016   133
S.A. Davis (ed.), *Adherence in Dermatology*,
DOI 10.1007/978-3-319-30994-1_12

to determine the numerous factors influencing adherence to protective measures that ward off sun damage.

Localized scleroderma is a connective tissue disorder which presents in three distinct forms: morphea, generalized morphea, and linear scleroderma [8]. Based upon the literature, the complexity of localized scleroderma indicates that intervention should be targeted based upon variation or subtype [9].

12.2   Methods

To better understand compliance behavior across these multiple areas of dermatology, we searched articles relating to sunscreen use/skin cancer, actinic keratosis, and localized scleroderma. PubMed was utilized as a search engine, with article publication dates ranging between the years 1987 and 2014. Search terms included adherence, sunscreen, skin cancer, actinic keratosis, and localized scleroderma. A table was created to ascertain adherence behavior with regard to prevention and treatment.

Target	Adherence type (preventative vs. treatment)	Intervention
(1) Skin cancer	Preventative	One-time education program
(2) Skin cancer; premature aging	Preventative	Appearance-based vs. health-based video
(3) Skin cancer	Preventative	Text message reminders
(4) Actinic keratosis	Treatment	N/A
(5) Actinic keratosis	Treatment	N/A
(6) Actinic keratosis	Treatment	N/A
(7) Localized scleroderma	Treatment	N/A

12.3   Results

1. The authors noted that Switzerland had a particularly high incidence of skin cancer relative to other countries in Europe; further, they cited excessive sun exposure during youth as a key contributing factor in the development of skin cancer [7]. Due to these reasons, the authors assayed the effectiveness of a school-based sun safety program on sun-related knowledge, protective actions, and sunburn rate on elementary school students [7]. An intervention was developed in which one hour education sessions on sun safety were implemented across 33 elementary schools; child participants included first, second, and third graders [7]. Via questionnaire, subjects answered inquiries regarding their sun-related knowledge, behaviors, and experience with sunburn; these questionnaires were administered before intervention and then again 1 year after intervention [7].

Researchers determined that 1 year after intervention, there was a statistically significant increase in sun-related knowledge; however, the findings did not suggest a similar trend in sun-protective behavior, such as sunscreen use [7].

2. The authors compared the effectiveness of appearance-based versus health-based video education in improving sunscreen knowledge and use [10]. Participants were 50 high-school students; the intervention occurred once, and subjects were randomly assigned to one of two groups [10]. One group of participants viewed a video which was appearance based (focused on UV-induced premature aging), while the other group watched a video which was health based (focused on the relationship between UV exposure and skin cancer) [10].

   For both appearance-based and health-based groups, there was a statistically significant increase in UV-related knowledge. In terms of behavior, for the health-based group, there was a nonsignificant increase in sunscreen use; however, a significant increase in sunscreen use was seen for the appearance-based group [10]. Further, the findings demonstrated that the appearance-based group applied sunscreen at significantly greater frequencies than did the health based [10].

3. To improve sunscreen adherence, and thus abate the risk of skin cancer development, researchers developed an intervention involving modern technology [11]. Specifically, a text messaging reminder was utilized as a way to improve compliance to daily sunscreen use [11]. Investigators performed a randomized, controlled trial on 70 subjects from the general community. Each participant owned a cellular phone containing text message features, and, importantly, they were able to retrieve text messages; subjects were also at least 18 years of age [11]. Two groups were devised from the participant pool: for a period of 6 weeks, half of the subjects received daily text reminders, while the other half did not [11]. From the 6-week study duration, the number of days in which subjects used sunscreen was used to measure sunscreen application adherence [11]. At baseline, there were no statistically significant differences between the two groups [11]. The participants who received daily text message reminders demonstrated a 56.1 % mean daily sunscreen adherence rate; in comparison, those who did not receive daily text reminders had a mean daily compliance rate of 30 % [11].

4. Actinic keratosis (AK) is a significant risk factor for squamous cell carcinoma; furthermore, AK is implicated as an early development stage of the mentioned carcinogenesis [12]. Although topical therapy is noted in the treatment of AK, there is insufficient research regarding the obstacles associated with such treatment [12]. The authors examined the challenges regarding adherence in those receiving topical therapy for actinic keratosis; they also explored perceptions of adherence and persistence which were included in their assay of real-world experience with topical therapies [12]. Physicians across eight countries completed a 45-min online survey [regarding topical therapy in treatment of actinic keratosis] [12]. Over half of the respondents agreed that topical field therapy was integral to AK treatment; additionally, the respondents' general consensus was that lengthy treatment duration and local skin reactions were key contributing factors to nonadherence/persistence in treatment [12]. A prescription involving the shortest duration in treatment would be preferred by more than 90 % of the physician respondents [12].

5. Topical 5-fluorouracil is recognized as an effective treatment for actinic keratosis; however, a lack of patient adherence seems to usurp this, and other type,
medication's value [13]. The authors note that, in terms of compliance assessment, electronic monitors provide more dependable data than do patient self-
reports; one reason for this discrepancy is that many individuals tend to
overestimate their treatment use [13]. In their study, adherence was assessed via
electronic monitors concealed in topical 5-fluorouracil, 0.5 %, cream medication
caps [13]. The study recruited 20 participants who presented with moderate to
severe face and scalp actinic keratosis [13]. A medication event monitoring system (MEMS) cap was attached to the fluorouracil, 0.5 %, cream provided to each
research subject [13]. For a 4-week period, participants were instructed to use
the treatment each evening [13]. Patient skin quality, local skin reaction, and
number of actinic keratosis lesions were measured at baseline and every 2 weeks
for an 8-week duration [13]. The study's electronic monitoring system demonstrated that adherence to the topical medication ranged from 54 to 100 %; overall, mean MEMS was 86 % and a reduction from 92 % at week 1 to 82 % at week
4 was observed over the 4-week active treatment period [13]. Interestingly,
results did not indicate that disease severity influenced adherence [13].
6. In the absence of surgical intervention, stringent adherence is required on the
part of the patient; additionally, choice of treatment is directly related to patient
perceptions of different potential treatments [14]. "Silent perspectives" that
patients held regarding treatment were explored via attention on individual user
viewpoints and experiences [14]. Twenty-four subjects participated in telephone
and face-to-face interviews; these were participants who had experienced treatment with one or more of the following therapies: 5-fluorouracil (5-FU) cream
5 %, diclofenac sodium gel 3 %, imiquimod 5 %, or photodynamic therapy [12].
Of major focus were efficiency of treatment, patient experience of pain, and
discharging ulcers; of lesser concern, yet still worth noting, were appearance,
social contacts, and leisure time [14]. Further, the perception that patients held in
terms of treatment instructions highlighted the risk of misinterpretation of directions [14]. Findings demonstrated that therapeutic efficiency was of primary
concern to patients [14].
7. The literature indicates that due to the complexity of localized scleroderma, interventions should be targeted to each variant of the disease [9]. The difficulty in
designing and testing an effective intervention for adherence for the subtypes of
localized scleroderma appears to live within the lack of evidence for optimal
treatment [15]. Although myriad topical and systemic regimens for therapy have
been suggested, the authors note that results of such treatment have been mixed
[15]. The researchers investigating potentially successful treatment for localized
scleroderma did, however, find evidence for an effective treatment of this disease
[15]. In their study, the authors suggested that clinical outcome is affected by both
dose and administration route of immunosuppressive regimens [15]. Through
their single-center localized scleroderma treatment protocol, they demonstrated
the effectiveness that a daily tapering dose of corticosteroids and parenteral methotrexate had on controlling the activity of localized scleroderma [15].

12.4 Discussion

There is an inextricable link between patient health and adherence to prescriber's recommendations [1]. Furthermore, the healthcare system suffers an economic upset as a result of noncompliant behavior [2]. This chapter has explored adherence in two manners, prevention and treatment, and across multiple areas of dermatology: sun-induced skin damage (with an emphasis on skin carcinogenesis, premature aging, and actinic keratosis) and localized scleroderma.

The results of the studies related to sun-induced skin damage, which presents in skin cancer, premature aging, and actinic keratosis, demonstrate some notable findings. Overall, it appears as though interventions designed to provide participants with information about the sun do increase subjects' knowledge; however, this does not necessarily translate into increased use of sunscreen and other protective measures [7, 10]. Interestingly, in one particular study (2), it did appear as though when the program was designed around appearance-based reasons to boost sun-protective behavior, a significant increase in sunscreen use was observed [10]. This finding reveals that interventions targeting the appearance-based reasons for sun-protective behavior might be effective in increasing sunscreen use, as well as other protective measures. A suggestion for further design development should include information related to both health and appearance. Markedly, two of the listed studies regarding skin cancer (1, 2) and premature aging (2) were carried out for only one session [7, 10]; given that one session of an informative program ostensibly increased sun-related knowledge across the board, it is possible that carrying these studies out for a longer duration might demonstrate an increase in sun-protective behavior, whether health or appearance based.

Another study which incorporated the use of modern technology, in the form of daily electronic text message reminders, demonstrated the effectiveness of their method [11]. A 26.1 % difference in compliance was seen between those study participants who received daily text reminders to their cellular telephones versus those who did not; with the group who experienced the electronic reminders showing greater adherence to daily sunscreen application [11]. This study is valuable in that it presents a way in which modern technology can be utilized in a cost-effective manner to improve patient adherence to daily sunscreen application [11]; if applied to a widespread audience, this intervention type has the potential to reduce skin cancer incidence.

Long-term exposure to the sun is implicated in the development of actinic keratosis, which presents as a scaly and coarse patch on the skin [4]. Actinic keratosis lesions are a major risk factor in the development of squamous cell carcinoma [12]. Studies on actinic keratosis seem to place a major focus on topical field therapy as treatment; furthermore, they include the possible adverse effects of such treatment and the lengthy persistence required as factors linked to nonadherence [12]. Patient perception of treatment for actinic keratosis is also seen as an important factor which contributes to adherence, with perception of therapeutic efficiency being of particular importance [14].

One study on actinic keratosis explored the value of an electronic monitoring system as a way to assess treatment adherence [13]. In this manner, an electronic monitoring system was not used as an intervention to increase medication compliance, but rather as a way to demonstrate the tool's usefulness in measuring such behavior. Although their research did not involve an intervention to necessarily improve compliance, it certainly provided valuable insight. The authors noted that patients seem to overestimate their medication use [13]. By including an electronic monitoring system that could allow patients to view their own behavior, thus holding them accountable, adherence might be improved.

Localized scleroderma is a complex disorder which requires differential intervention depending on type [9]. The research regarding this particular condition notes the lack of evidence for an optimal course of treatment, despite the range of therapeutic options [15]. However, in their single-center study of localized scleroderma, researchers noted the effects of both administration route and dose of immunosuppressive regimens [15]. Moreover, the authors determined that a daily dose tapering of corticosteroids and parenteral methotrexate had a beneficial effect on managing the action of localized scleroderma [15]. It seems clear that in order to determine methods to increase adherence in the treatment of localized scleroderma, more attention needs to be paid to research substantiating effective therapeutic regimens.

As the information in this chapter has demonstrated, there are myriad factors which contribute to adherence and nonadherence, in terms of both prevention and treatment. The discussed intervention strategies – such as patient education (especially appealing to concern with appearance), frequent electronic contact, and choosing a sensible dose and administration route – offer valuable insight into the ways in which future research can work to enhance therapeutic outcomes. Both patient health and the medical community suffer as a result of noncompliance [1, 2]. It is therefore of critical value that we continue to explore ideas and interventions that have the potential to improve adherence.

References

1. Lee IA, Maibach HI (2006) Pharmionics in dermatology: a review of topical medication adherence. Am J Clin Dermatol 7(4):231–236
2. Osterberg L, Blaschke T (2005) Adherence to medication. N Engl J Med 353:487–497
3. Cho H, Lee S, Wilson K (2010) Magazine exposure, tanned women stereotypes, and tanning attitudes. Body Image 7(4):364–367
4. Nolan BV, Feldman SR (2009) Ultraviolet tanning addiction. Dermatol Clin 27(2):109–112
5. Mancebo SE, Hu JY, Wang SQ (2014) Sunscreens: a review of health benefits, regulations, and controversies. Dermatol Clin 32(3):427–438
6. Rogers HW, Weinstock MA, Feldman SR, Coldiron BM (2015) Incidence estimate of nonmelanoma skin cancer (keratinocyte carcinomas) in the U.S. Population. JAMA Dermatol 151(10):1081–1086
7. Reinau D, Meier CR, Gerber N, Surber C (2014) Evaluation of a sun safety education programme for primary school students in Switzerland. Eur J Cancer Prev 23(4):303–309

8. Jackson CT, Maibach HI (2014) Localized scleroderma variants: pharmacologic implications. J Dermatol Treat 25(6):529–531
9. Fett N (2013) Scleroderma: nomenclature, etiology, pathogenesis, prognosis, and treatments: facts and controversies. Clin Dermatol 31(4):432–437
10. Tuong W, Armstrong AW (2014) Effect of appearance-based education compared with health-based education on sunscreen use and knowledge: a randomized controlled trial. J Am Acad Dermatol 70(4):665–669
11. Armstrong AW, Watson AJ, Makredes M, Frangos JE, Kimball AB, Kvedar JC (2009) Text-message reminders to improve sunscreen use: a randomized, controlled trial using electronic monitoring. Arch Dermatol 145(11):1230–1236
12. Stockfleth E, Peris K, Guillen C, Cerio R, Basset-Seguin N, Foley P, Sanches J, Culshaw A, Erntoft S, Lebwohl M (2015) Physician perceptions and experience of current treatment in actinic keratosis. J Eur Acad Dermatol Venereol 29(2):298–306
13. Yentzer B, Hick J, Williams L, Inabinet R, Wilson R, Camacho FT, Russell GB, Feldman SR (2009) Adherence to a topical regimen of 5-fluorouracil, 0.5%, cream for the treatment of actinic keratoses. Arch Dermatol 145(2):203–205
14. Esmann S, Jemec GB (2014) Patients' perceptions of topical treatments of actinic keratosis. J Dermatol Treat 25(5):375–379
15. Torok KS, Arkachaisri T (2012) Methotrexate and corticosteroids in the treatment of localized scleroderma: a standardized prospective longitudinal single-center study. J Rheumatol 39(2):286–294

Part IV
Strategies to Improve Adherence

Chapter 13
Optimizing the Physician-Patient Relationship and Educating the Patient About Adherence

Scott A. Davis and Steven R. Feldman

Optimizing the physician-patient relationship is perhaps the most fundamental piece of the adherence challenge. Physicians who evoke feelings of trust, confidence, and empathy from their patients are more likely to observe good patient adherence [1]. Although the term "compliance," based on a paternalistic view of the clinical encounter, is now considered outdated, the regimen is still suggested by the physician more often than not. Patients who want to please their physician are likely to be more willing to make an honest attempt to perform the treatment regimen correctly. Starting off well, and consequently seeing early improvement in disease, is likely to lead to higher satisfaction and long-term adherence [1, 2]. In contrast, patients with negative feelings toward their physician are likely to be more influenced by fears, temporary setbacks (such as side effects), and gradual loss of patience with the regimen, which are all major reasons for poor adherence and early discontinuation. Trust is also a two-way street, influencing the reliability of communication from the patient to the physician as well [3]. With a better rapport, it is more likely that patients will honestly admit areas of concern, and physicians will gain better information to produce good decisions.

S.A. Davis (✉)
Department of Dermatology, Wake Forest School of Medicine, Winston-Salem, NC, USA

Division of Pharmaceutical Outcomes and Policy, University of North Carolina Eshelman School of Pharmacy, Chapel Hill, NC, USA
e-mail: sdavis81@email.unc.edu

S.R. Feldman
Departments of Dermatology, Pathology, and Public Health Sciences,
Wake Forest School of Medicine, Winston-Salem, NC, USA

© Springer International Publishing Switzerland 2016   143
S.A. Davis (ed.), *Adherence in Dermatology*,
DOI 10.1007/978-3-319-30994-1_13

13.1 Service Excellence: Understanding What Patients Perceive as a "Good Doctor"

In a variety of studies using data from the physician rating website DrScore.com, physician empathy consistently rated as by far the most important factor [4]. Patients who had a long wait still tended to give ratings of 10 out of 10, provided they felt they had seen a caring, empathetic doctor. The top predictor of patient adherence in one study was when patients viewed their physicians as compassionate advocates [5]. In addition, patients who are asked for their feedback tend to be more pleased; measuring patient satisfaction inevitably changes patient satisfaction [6]. Physicians can then view their own ratings and find out what aspects of the care they offer is appreciated (providing positive reinforcement) and what seemed potentially unsatisfactory to patients and can be improved.

Many physicians are surprised to find that their technical competence goes relatively unappreciated in patient satisfaction surveys, since it is hard for lay people to understand the thought processes in the physician's brain, potentially leading to miscommunication. For example, a physician who diagnosed psoriasis in just a split second, based on recognition of common patterns from years of intense dermatology training, might make a negative impression on the patient [3]. Instead of coming across as incredibly technically competent, this type of physician might seem not to have done a thorough exam and might strike the patient as uncaring [3]. Even after making the rapid diagnosis, the physician may take time to do a few things that make patients realize a thorough examination was done, including looking at the psoriasis closely and touching the lesions, combating the stigma that psoriasis patients inevitably experience. For a lesion that might be malignant, looking at it closely under a magnifying glass would send the right message that a careful examination was done, even though the real decision will be made as a result of a biopsy or, in the case of obvious lesions, may have been made from across the room [3].

13.2 Educating the Patient

Educating patients about adherence has many facets, including transmission of knowledge and skills, assessment and clarification of values, and persuasive health communication. Knowledge and skills would include how to store and administer the medication correctly, including when to take it as well as technique for how to inject biologics or apply topicals. Assessment and clarification of values involves situations where different patients may have different preferences, but a range of choices is still clinically reasonable. For example, patients with different levels of risk tolerance may have different preferences among biologics, methotrexate, or phototherapy for severe psoriasis treatment. Finally, persuasive health communication is required when clinical equipoise does not exist – when there is definitely a course of action that would be more beneficial than another, and the expert must communicate clinical knowledge persuasively to elicit better health behavior. Typical examples outside of dermatology include patients who smoke, drink too much alcohol, or engage in unsafe sex. A dermatological example might be a patient who has already had skin cancer yet continues to resist the need for sun protection.

According to the International Patient Decision Aid Standards (IPDAS), values clarification involves helping patients to prioritize the most important attributes of a health decision that influence their preference among available choices [7], such as which medication to take. Values clarification methods are processes that facilitate at least one of the following [7]:

1. Identifying options
2. Understanding how the patient's preferences affect the choice in the context of specific options and a specific situation
3. Reasoning about options or their characteristics
4. Using compensatory and/or non-compensatory decision rules to bring together information about various properties of different options (e.g., a sun-protective hat is very convenient and less expensive in the long term, but sunscreen potentially provides greater sun protection factor, so how does this patient feel about the relative importance of these attributes?)
5. Comparing options holistically
6. Retrieving values from long-term memory

Values clarification methods are considered most helpful when they evoke the most helpful mental representation (e.g., as described below in Communicating Risk), include consideration of all appropriate options, inhibit patients from hastily seizing on the first option considered, enhance recall of all important values from memory, assist in weighing the importance of various values, and allow plenty of time to make a final decision [8].

Persuasive health communication can be targeted – developed for a specific audience – or even tailored to a specific individual [9, 10]. An example of a tailored smoking cessation message involved materials in which a role model very similar to the patient provided a message of encouragement with specific answers to concerns that the patient had [11]. The role model was a person who had quit smoking recently and was matched to the patient on factors such as stage of change, age, gender, ethnicity, marital status, children, job status, and barriers [11]. The message included a picture of the role model and answers to the questions "Why did you decide to quit?", "How did you prepare for the change?", "Did you try anything else as your quit day approached?", "Did these things help?", and "Did you ask for help?" [11]. This example demonstrates the power of sharing advice that is perceived to originate from a peer, rather than a medical professional who might seem to be pushing an agenda to some degree. More information about persuasion is presented in Chap. 16.

13.2.1 Communicating Risk

Many patients are unwilling to take medications because of fear of side effects or toxicity related to overuse. One way to understand how patients think about risk and process information about treatments from clinicians is fuzzy-trace theory. Fuzzy-trace theory suggests that patients tend to keep two separate representations in memory of any statement they have heard: a verbatim representation and a gist representation [12, 13]. Recollection of the gist representation tends to be prioritized in decision making, so it is important to communicate information in such a way that the right gist representation will be retained. Perhaps surprisingly, decision making based on gist processing is considered a more developmentally advanced form of decision making, which adults and subject-matter experts prefer more strongly than children and nonexperts [14]. Despite occasional errors that might be avoidable by using the verbatim representation, gist-based decision making performs well enough that people grow to prefer it.

Unfortunately, since different listeners encode gist representations of the same material in different ways, clinicians can never be sure that they are transmitting the exact gist they intended. However, trying to minimize the number of distinct messages in a communication may enhance recall. Also, anticipate problems when there is a very salient message that would tend to overwhelm the rest of the communication, especially what comes after the salient message. For example, if patients are told they have cancer, they generally fixate on that very distressing fact and have poor recall of anything communicated in the subsequent part of the visit.

Returning to fear of medications, a common situation in which patients develop excessive fear is when a relative risk is presented, even though the absolute difference in risk is very small. Patients might hear that severe psoriasis doubles their risk of a heart attack, whereas the absolute risk of heart attack for patients in their 40s with severe psoriasis is still only 1 in 600 [15]. The risk of inflammatory bowel disease (IBD) for patients taking isotretinoin might sound scary if presented as a doubling of risk, whereas if it is presented as an increase from 1 in 10,000 to 2 in 10,000, it is more evident that the risk difference is only 0.0001 (it may be perceived as even safer if presented as "9,998 out of 10,000 don't develop IBD"). Another way to present the same information is as a number needed to treat (NNT), which is 1 divided by the absolute value of the risk difference. If the risk difference is 0.0001, the NNT is 10,000, indicating that 10,000 additional patients would have to be treated with isotretinoin to cause 1 additional IBD case. A way to communicate this information graphically is to show an appropriate image such as a basketball arena packed with 20,000 fans for a big game, but with only two people highlighted. This image vividly conveys the fact that if everyone in the arena were treated with isotretinoin, only two additional people would be expected to get IBD (assuming there is a twofold risk caused by isotretinoin; whether there is any true increased risk of IBD due to isotretinoin is unclear), in addition to the two people who would get IBD without treatment.

The concept of anchoring in behavioral economics also suggests a way to communicate small risks more effectively. By saying, "The risk of side effects with this medication is greater than that of a lightning strike," the lightning strike is used as an anchor – in this case, a very rare event that provides a reference point for comparison [16]. If a higher anchor were used, such as, "The risk of side effects with this medication is less than that of a coin flip," a very different message would be communicated, suggesting that the risk was similar to that of a common event.

Although it is helpful to communicate risks graphically and by using anchors, many patients still assign disproportionate weight to very small risks. People act approximately the same way in response to a 1/100,000 risk as they do to a 1/1,000 risk [17, 18], such as by being just as likely to buy the same amount of insurance against both risks. As predicted by fuzzy-trace theory, people's gist representation of both risks might be identical ("a small risk") but greatly different from that of a zero risk. If a patient is fixated on the risk of one treatment, suggesting another treatment that does not have that risk – even though it has other risks – may relieve the patient's concern. It may also be helpful to emphasize that there is no truly risk-free strategy; avoiding treatment and continuing to suffer from the disease also has risks [16]. For example, if a patient is obese due to a sedentary lifestyle exacerbated by disabling psoriasis, the risk reduction in serious health consequences achieved by successful biologic treatment of psoriasis may exceed the risk of the medication. By dissuading the patient from an initial frame of a risky course of action vs. a risk-free course of action and instead arguing that either possible action has some risk, it may be possible to elicit a more rational choice.

13.2.2 Written Action Plans

Written action plans are available for several chronic conditions that often necessitate complex regimens, such as atopic dermatitis [19] and psoriasis [3]. Giving clear written instructions is essential since patients are not likely to recall details of complex regimens, such as atopic dermatitis regimens involving wet wraps in addition to topical corticosteroids and moisturizers. Prepare preprinted educational materials and keep them in each exam room ready to hand out [3]. These materials are often available from patient advocacy organizations such as the National Psoriasis Foundation.

13.3 Special Issues: Adolescents

Adolescents typically show one of the lowest adherence rates of any age group [20]. Adolescents have a low tolerance for delayed gratification and also are often in conflict with parents [1]. Parents often demand that something be done, but the adolescent is typically more interested in asserting independence, even if it means continuing to have the disease [3]. In one study, teenagers whose parents received

Table 13.1 Strategies to improve adolescents' adherence

Encourage development of adolescents' self-management skills, rather than dependence on others for ensuring adherence [22–24]
Spend some time meeting with the adolescent one-on-one, without the parent in the room, unless the adolescent spontaneously states they would prefer to have the parent present [1]
Direct conversation toward the adolescent to communicate the message that the adolescent (not the parent) is the patient [1]
Win the respect of the adolescent by refuting myths that the parent might believe (such as that eating too many French fries causes acne) [1]
Understand the adolescent's lifestyle (e.g., sports played, cosmetics used) and assist in choosing a non-messy vehicle that accommodates that lifestyle [1]
Involve the adolescent in the choice of treatment, including vehicle and schedule (morning vs. evening use) [1]
Understand when patients do not want to be treated (scores below 5 on a 1–10 scale of how much the disease affects them), and do not try to force them to get treated [1]
Understand the norms of the adolescent's peer group, e.g., whether taking medication is viewed as acceptable by friends [23]
Appeal to conformity by saying that a medication is what other adolescents use to have control of their condition [3]
Tailor the level of parental reminding behavior to the amount of supervision that the adolescent wants; rein in overzealous parents [3]
Be sure to ask open-ended questions about side effects and how well the medications are working [25]
Consider using apps that allow documentation of medication history and sharing medication use information with the provider [26]

daily phone calls to remind the teenagers to take acne medications were less adherent than the control group [21].

Recognizing that the adolescent's own motivation has primary importance, and respecting the adolescent's need for independence, some special strategies for improving adolescents' adherence can be employed (Table 13.1). In a series of studies on diseases ranging from diabetes to juvenile rheumatoid arthritis (JRA), Kyngas and colleagues defined several key components that adolescents ages 13–17 viewed as essential for encouraging their medication adherence [22, 23]. Based on adolescents' own stated perceptions, Kyngas classified physician behaviors as motivating, authoritarian, inattentive, routine, or a combination of inattentive and routine [23]. Diabetic patients whose physicians acted in a motivating style were by far the most adherent, whereas physicians who were both inattentive and routine elicited the worst adherence [23]. When a routine style was used, adolescents complained that the physician did not care about them as individuals and only talked, without listening [23]. In a later study, Kyngas assessed perceived physician support according to the reports of adolescent patients with asthma, epilepsy, diabetes, or JRA [22]. Adolescents perceived good physician support and had consequent higher adherence when physicians scored high in the following domains: (1) "paying attention to my life situation and problems when planning my treatment", (2) "showing interest in me not only my disease", (3) "not ordering how I should act", and (4) "encouraging me to take care of myself" [22].

13.4 Conclusion

Generating good rapport and trust creates a foundation for addressing each patient's unique adherence issues. Good communication ensures that patients can disclose their adherence barriers honestly so that each barrier can be addressed. Careful attention to nonverbal messages increases the chance of sending the right message about the clinician's commitment to service and caring. Risk communication can be enhanced by applying tactics to overcome the cognitive limitations suggested by behavioral economics and fuzzy-trace theory. In the next few chapters, we will look at how to reap the benefits of a strong, trusting relationship as we turn to strategies for choosing the right treatment, dealing with forgetfulness, and building motivation and self-efficacy.

References

1. Baldwin HE (2006) Tricks for improving compliance with acne therapy. Dermatol Ther 19(4):224–236
2. Feldman SR, Horn EJ, Balkrishnan R et al (2008) Psoriasis: improving adherence to topical therapy. J Am Acad Dermatol 59(6):1009–1016
3. Feldman SR (2009) Practical ways to improve patients' treatment outcomes. Medical Quality Enhancement Corporation, Winston-Salem
4. Uhas AA, Camacho FT, Feldman SR, Balkrishnan R (2008) The relationship between physician friendliness and caring, and patient satisfaction: findings from an internet-based survey. Patient 1(2):91–96
5. Felkey BG (1995) Adherence screening and monitoring. Am Pharm NS35(7):42–51; quiz 52–53
6. Glenn C, McMichael A, Feldman SR (2012) Measuring patient satisfaction changes patient satisfaction. J Dermatol Treat 23(2):81–82
7. Fagerlin A, Pignone M, Abhyankar P et al (2013) Clarifying values: an updated review. BMC Med Informat Decis Making 13(Suppl 2):S8
8. Pieterse AH, de Vries M, Kunneman M, Stiggelbout AM, Feldman-Stewart D (2013) Theory-informed design of values clarification methods: a cognitive psychological perspective on patient health-related decision making. Soc Sci Med 77:156–163
9. Noar SM, Harrington NG, Van Stee SK, Aldrich RS (2011) Tailored health communication to change lifestyle behaviors. Am J Lifestyle Med 5:112–122
10. Rimer BK, Kreuter MW (2006) Advancing tailored health communication: a persuasion and message effects perspective. J Commun 56:S184–S201
11. Strecher VJ, McClure J, Alexander G et al (2008) The role of engagement in a tailored web-based smoking cessation program: randomized controlled trial. J Med Internet Res 10(5):e36
12. Reyna VF (2004) How people make decisions that involve risk: a dual-processes approach. Curr Dir Psychol Sci 13(2):60–66
13. Blalock SJ, Slota C, Devellis BM et al (2014) Patient-rheumatologist communication concerning prescription medications: getting to the gist. Arthritis Care Res 66(4):542–550
14. Reyna VF, Lloyd FJ (2006) Physician decision making and cardiac risk: effects of knowledge, risk perception, risk tolerance, and fuzzy processing. J Exp Psychol Appl 12(3):179–195
15. Gelfand JM, Neimann AL, Shin DB, Wang X, Margolis DJ, Troxel AB (2006) Risk of myocardial infarction in patients with psoriasis. JAMA 296(14):1735–1741
16. Davis SA, Feldman SR (2014) An illustrated dictionary of behavioral economics for healthcare professionals. CreateSpace, Charleston

17. Sunstein CR (2002) Probability neglect: emotions, worst cases, and law. Yale Law J 112:61–107
18. Rottenstreich Y, Hsee CK (2001) Money, kisses, and electric shocks: on the affective psychology of risk. Psychol Sci 12(3):185–190
19. Ntuen E, Taylor SL, Kinney M, O'Neill JL, Krowchuk DP, Feldman SR (2010) Physicians' perceptions of an eczema action plan for atopic dermatitis. J Dermatol Treat 21(1):28–33
20. DiMatteo MR (2004) Variations in patients' adherence to medical recommendations: a quantitative review of 50 years of research. Med Care 42(3):200–209
21. Yentzer BA, Gosnell AL, Clark AR et al (2011) A randomized controlled pilot study of strategies to increase adherence in teenagers with acne vulgaris. J Am Acad Dermatol 64(4):793–795
22. Kyngas H, Rissanen M (2001) Support as a crucial predictor of good compliance of adolescents with a chronic disease. J Clin Nurs 10(6):767–774
23. Kyngas H, Hentinen M, Barlow JH (1998) Adolescents' perceptions of physicians, nurses, parents and friends: help or hindrance in compliance with diabetes self-care? J Adv Nurs 27(4):760–769
24. Drotar D (2009) Physician behavior in the care of pediatric chronic illness: association with health outcomes and treatment adherence. J Dev Behav Pediatr JDBP 30(3):246–254
25. Sleath B, Carpenter DM, Ayala GX et al (2011) Provider discussion, education, and question-asking about control medications during pediatric asthma visits. Int J Pediatr 2011:212160
26. Bailey SC, Belter LT, Pandit AU, Carpenter DM, Carlos E, Wolf MS (2014) The availability, functionality, and quality of mobile applications supporting medication self-management. J Am Med Inform Assoc JAMIA 21(3):542–546

Chapter 14
Choosing the Treatment the Patient Is Most Likely To Use

Dennis A. Hopkinson, Andrew J. Huang, Karen E. Huang, and Steven R. Feldman

As clinicians who treat skin disorders, a dilemma dermatologists face when devising a treatment regimen is choosing among several, sometimes dozens of, medications that vary in their efficacy and safety profile, all of which may be appropriate treatments to use. Although there may be a plethora of good treatment options, many patients who are prescribed these treatments will continue to show evidence of disease, often as a result of poor adherence. The goal of this chapter is to first provide an overview on the fundamentals of patient adherence and then to delve into the literature regarding the optimization of four aspects of treatment selection: matters regarding convenience, drug vehicles, treatment efficacy, and preferences regarding adverse effects. The definitive goal is to arrive at a personalized, convenient, tolerable treatment to which the patient is most likely to adhere.

14.1 Fundamentals of Selecting the Appropriate Treatment

14.1.1 Building the Relationship

The first step of formulating the optimal treatment plan for a patient is an open and honest discussion that explores the patient's views and preferences, as these discussions not only help determine the most appropriate treatment but also inherently increase patient satisfaction and treatment adherence [1, 2]. These gains in treatment

D.A. Hopkinson, MD • A.J. Huang, MD • K.E. Huang, MS
Department of Dermatology, Wake Forest School of Medicine, Winston-Salem, NC, USA
e-mail: keaanensen@gmail.com

S.R. Feldman, MD, PhD (✉)
Departments of Dermatology, Pathology, and Public Health Sciences, Wake Forest School of Medicine, Winston-Salem, NC, USA
e-mail: sfeldman@wakehealth.edu

© Springer International Publishing Switzerland 2016
S.A. Davis (ed.), *Adherence in Dermatology*,
DOI 10.1007/978-3-319-30994-1_14

Table 14.1 Key discussion points in this chapter

Section	Key points discussed
Fundamentals of selecting the appropriate treatment	The physician-patient relationship, reasons for deliberate nonadherence and methods used to address this challenge, rotational therapy
Convenience	Interactions with food, location of treatment, duration of treatment, number of daily doses, radiotherapy, acne treatment
Vehicle	Layering, vehicle selection specific for teenagers and psoriasis, miscellaneous aspects of vehicle selection
Efficacy	Perceptions of efficacy, effect of living situation and age, combination therapy
Adverse effects	Trade-offs for benefit, demographic aspects, severity of skin disease, comorbidities, steroid phobia

adherence stem from patients feeling empowered when they are invited to participate in designing a treatment plan [1].The goal during these discussions is to match the patient's preferences to the dermatologist's knowledge of the relative efficacies of various therapies as well as to build rapport, with the ultimate aim of devising a treatment plan that is convenient, comfortable, effective, and minimally toxic (Table 14.1).

14.1.2   Deliberate Nonadherence

In dermatology, the primary reasons for deliberate nonadherence (as opposed to nondeliberate nonadherence, such as forgetfulness) are dissatisfaction with a treatment's perceived efficacy, inconvenience of the treatment, and side effects (as well as fear of potential side effects)—all matters that are important to address in the initial consultation [3]. One such example of a treatment that requires careful counseling is the use of isotretinoin in the treatment of cystic acne. Isotretinoin presents many potential hurdles to adherence: the initial worsening of a patient's acne that could be interpreted as a failure of the medication; the drug being best taken with meals, which could be inconvenient for those on atypical eating schedules or who eat in groups; overt skin peeling which may cause additional stress to patients who are concerned about their current appearance, even if the patient understands that the peeling is a sign that the medication is beginning to work; having to navigate the iPLEDGE system; and the general gestalt that isotretinoin is scary stuff [4].

14.1.3   Rotational Therapy

Another example of a treatment regimen where patients are likely to deliberately non-adhere is "rotational therapy," where medications with significant adverse effects are rotated on a periodic basis. The purpose of rotation therapy is to cycle

Table 14.2 Key aspects of consideration when selecting a treatment regimen	Important considerations when selecting an appropriate treatment plan
	Location of treatment (home, physician's office, inpatient)
	Mode of delivery (topical, oral, phototherapy, injection)
	Side effects and willingness to trade side effects for efficacy and rapid results
	Preferred "feel" of topical application
	Desired degree of benefit
	Patient lifestyle and want for convenience

through several medications with different associated toxicities in order to spread the cumulative toxicity to multiple organ sites [5]. Physicians who treat pain, for example, often employ this method on a short time scale by alternating acetaminophen and ibuprofen to minimize cumulative renal and hepatic toxicity. In dermatology, rotational therapy has been employed in the treatment of severe atopic dermatitis and psoriasis, whereby medications such as ultraviolet light therapy, coal tar, methotrexate, cyclosporine, and high-potency topical steroids were rotated on a scale of months to years (note: the need for rotational therapy in psoriasis has been greatly reduced by highly effective, safer biologic treatments) [5, 6].

Unfortunately, patients are often reluctant to switch medication regimens and may prefer to stay on one treatment if they find that it suits them [7]. Knowing this, it is beneficial to emphasize during patient counseling that rotational therapy is integral in minimizing the long-term probability of renal failure (cyclosporine), skin cancer (UVA and UVB light therapy), skin thinning (topical corticosteroids), and infections (TNF inhibitors). If rotation therapy is indeed the most appropriate treatment, it may be possible to increase a patient's openness to this approach by indicating that rotational therapy is readily customizable—should the next therapy in the rotation be intolerable or less efficacious, adjustments can be made (Table 14.2).

14.2   Convenience

14.2.1   Interactions with Food

Several medications used in the treatment of acne have interactions with food and will be rendered less effective or result in adverse effects if the directions are not followed. For example, isotretinoin is a fat-soluble retinoid that is best absorbed when taken with meals, especially meals that have some degree of fat content. This can be a difficult task for a teenager who eats breakfast and lunch away from home or in the presence of their peers as they may feel embarrassed by taking a pill with friends around [8]. A patient who is currently in an extended period of fasting, as may happen for religious observations, may also be a poor candidate for isotretinoin. Another poor candidate would be a patient who adheres to a low-fat diet—this subset of patients would benefit from the formulation of isotretinoin that does not rely on fat in the gastrointestinal tract for absorption [9].

On the opposite end of the spectrum, tetracycline is a water-soluble antibiotic that interacts with multiple foods and chelates several minerals including calcium, thereby losing its potency if taken on a full stomach, with multivitamins or with dairy products [8, 10]. These properties make it difficult for patients who enjoy intermittent snacks or have a high dairy intake to adhere to this drug, and thus choosing an antibiotic less prone to these effects would be advised. Doxycycline and minocycline have weak interactions with certain foods, but clindamycin and trimethoprim/sulfamethoxazole are safe to take with or without food.

14.2.2   Location of Treatment

Patients often have strong feelings about the location of their treatment and usually prioritize their preferences in the following order: at home, at an outpatient clinic, and, finally, as an inpatient [11]. An example of a treatment that can be administered in both the home and clinic setting is phototherapy. It is more convenient for a patient to receive phototherapy at home versus at a facility, and as a result, compliance levels are high with home treatment [12]; unfortunately, though the overall cost of home phototherapy makes it highly cost effective, the out-of-pocket cost of a home phototherapy device to a patient can be prohibitively expensive. Patients with psoriasis who must attend a treatment facility often have to weigh the cost/ benefit ratio of three times a week versus two times a week phototherapy. While it can be inconvenient to travel three times a week for treatment, more rapid results can be achieved with three times per week treatment phototherapy compared to two times per week treatment, and some patients prefer the increased speed to remission at the expense of convenience. Thus it is reasonable to bring these options up in conversation [13].

While inpatient therapy may be both costly and inconvenient, there are still patient subgroups that benefit from hospitalization or intensive outpatient treatment programs. Patients with severe psoriasis who are refractory to therapy, who are retired or unemployed, and who like the idea of regularly attending outpatient care would be ideal candidates for a multi-week Goeckerman regimen of tar and ultraviolet light therapy or an Ingram regimen of anthralin paste added to the Goeckerman regimen [14]. Several hospitals in the United States now offer Goeckerman therapy at day units, lowering the cost of therapy compared to hospitalization. While the level of disease that warrants an inpatient stay is uncommon, hospitalization can be beneficial in that it is a technique that ensures adherence to highly effective therapy.

14.2.3   Length of Treatments

The time required to administer a single treatment is another aspect to consider when choosing a modality of therapy. Office-based UV treatments are not only inconvenient in that they may require the patient to attend a certain location, but they also require a significant amount of time spent in the treatment center. The alternative, topical therapies, can be time consuming and bothersome—26 % of patients using topical treatments for psoriasis report poor adherence as a result of the length of time required to apply the topical agent [15]. For patients with psoriasis, longer treatment durations were associated with lower adherence rates [16, 17]. As a result, shortening treatment lengths can improve patient adherence, and patients should be educated on how long they can expect a course of treatment will be. From a psychological perspective, patients are more amenable to adhering to a plan for a shorter duration. An example of this can be found in the successful Alcoholics Anonymous program which emphasizes a short time horizon with the phrase "just for today" [18].

14.2.4   Frequency of Treatment

The number of times a patient must take a medication per day is inversely correlated to treatment adherence. In a cardiovascular observational study, adherence levels for antihypertensive medications were 84 % when a patient is on once-daily dosing, while patients on twice- or three-times-daily dose regimens took their medication on only 75 % and 59 % of days, respectively [19].

While once-daily dosing provides better adherence than more frequent dosing schedules, injectable medications can reduce the number of doses per day even lower. With etanercept, for example, capable patients can self-administer subcutaneous injections twice weekly for a period of 3 months [20]. This treatment regimen is also convenient in that it does not require travel for administration and requires little time to administer. While injectables do require refrigeration and periodic laboratory monitoring, patients are highly satisfied with the general ease of use of these agents and are significantly more satisfied with their treatment when compared to light therapy and oral therapy [20]. However, even with biologics adherence can be poor; thus, if a patient is interested in commencing an injectable treatment, adherence, results, and satisfaction should be monitored [21]. For patients with several medications, combining separate medications in a single tube or tablet effectively reduces the number of medications being taken each day and results in greater satisfaction and adherence [22–24].

14.2.5   Specifics Regarding Acne

Regarding topical applications, several interesting findings from a crossover study of multiple acne medications emerged, most regarding topical medications. Room temperature storage capability, a long product shelf life of 18 months or more, and the ability to apply with fingers as opposed to pad or other applicators are significantly preferable to patients [25]. Additionally, teenagers appreciate the convenience of individually packaged pledgets for the treatment of acne, as they can be carried around in an athletic bag or backpack [26]. Also, medicated cleaning cloths are preferred to washes for topicals in terms of convenience [27]. Another hurdle to adherence in acne is the complexity of the treatment regimen; simplifying the treatment regimen with products that contain multiple drugs can reduce treatment complexity and increase adherence [22]. Adherence can also be improved in patients with acne through the use of weekly online reporting of treatment progress [28].

14.3   Vehicle

The vehicles by which topical medications are administered influence patient satisfaction and adherence [29]. With options ranging from ointments, creams, lotions, gels, foams, mousses, and shampoos, it can be overwhelming to both the patient and the new physician when faced with choosing a "best" option. While there are no fixed definitions of the various types of vehicles, there are generally typical characteristics of the most common vehicles applicable to specific patient situations, and these can be discussed with patients.

14.3.1   Layering

Some patients dislike layering topical products, more so on the face and more so for daytime use. This preference was especially true for patients who intended on wearing makeup, sunscreens, and/or moisturizers [30]. To remedy this and avoid the problem of layers altogether, physicians can prescribe combination products to be applied in the evenings such as adapalene/benzoyl peroxide for acne or calcipotriene/betamethasone for psoriasis. If nighttime therapy is not an option, gels should be avoided in women who wear makeup as gels with high polymer concentrations can cause "beading up" of makeup [10]. Instead, lotions are recommended as they tend not to impede makeup application and can be applied to both oily and dry skin types [26].

14.3.2 Teenagers

Teenagers, especially boys, may dislike moisturizing vehicles such as creams and ointments and instead prefer gel or foam preparations [30]. Most teens do not mind using washes or masks and are likely to use them [30]. While not specific to teenagers, patients with oily skin and acne prefer gels because of the drying effect from the evaporation of the vehicle [10, 25]. Furthermore, minimizing visible side effects is highly valued by teenagers [30]. Because of these preferences, the use of vehicles with microsphere technology may be a consideration for teens to reduce visible side effects, which may improve adherence [30–33].

14.3.3 Psoriasis

Although ointments are an effective vehicle for corticosteroids due to their occlusive nature and lubricating qualities, patients with psoriasis generally prefer less messy vehicles such as foam and solution preparations over traditional cream and ointment vehicles [34]. Even though patients often prefer foams and creams over ointments, prescribing an ointment for nighttime use as monotherapy for mild psoriasis may be an option for some patients as ointments may be better tolerated at night and are very effective due to their occlusive and lubricating properties (though in one study patients reported disliking ointments as much at night as during the day) [35, 36].

Questioning the patient at follow-up visits regarding their satisfaction with the "feel" of each topical medication can be helpful when a clinician suspects nonadherence due to unwanted vehicle effects. Unfortunately, switching products to obtain a different vehicle can be costly. For example, trade named clobetasol propionate foam or shampoo can cost more than ten times than the equivalent generic ointment or cream if the patient lacks insurance coverage (the availability of coupons and the rapidly changing price of generics notwithstanding) [37–39]. Discussion regarding insurance status and financial stressors is appropriate in these settings as most pharmaceutical companies offer patient assistance programs to low-income or uninsured patients to offset the high out-of-pocket costs.

14.4 Efficacy

Efficacy of a medication is a key consideration when selecting a treatment regimen [15]. One of the primary reasons patients stop using their medication is a perceived lack of drug efficacy [15]. With regard to the durability of a treatment, those who had been suffering with chronic skin diseases for greater than 10 years and those who had been treated with more than three distinct treatments were more likely to be concerned about long-lasting benefits from their therapies [40].

14.4.1   Effect of Living Situation and Age

The relative importance of the efficacy of a treatment also varies with the demographics of a patient. Patients who are single place more emphasis on probability of benefit compared to those who are living with a partner [1]. Younger patients and women are highly interested in the probability of improvement of a treatment, while older patients (those greater than 65 years of age) are generally less concerned about the probability of improvement compared to other aspects of treatment [1].

14.4.2   Combination Therapy

One method of improving treatment results is through combination therapy, especially when the therapy is combined in a single tube or tablet, as mentioned above. Combination therapy results in greater efficacy and a more rapid outcome and an increase in adherence [41, 42].

14.4.3   Biologics

For those with psoriasis, another method of improving efficacy is by switching to an injectable biologic treatment, as satisfaction is higher in patients who are prescribed such medications as alefacept, etanercept, and infliximab compared to patients who are prescribed methotrexate, phototherapy, retinoids, and cyclosporine [20]. Not only were these drugs effective, patients also appreciated the convenience of the injection (see Sect. 14.2 above) [20].

14.5   Side Effects and Patient Choice

14.5.1   Generalities in Patient Priorities

When considering treatment side effects, many patients are most concerned about the risk of severe side effects and are less concerned about mild tolerability issues [43]. Still, some patients are willing to trade an increased risk of adverse events for increased probability and magnitude of benefit [44]. One potential difference in these viewpoints may be the result of the clinician fully describing severe adverse events to patients [1]. If the physician is to describe such rare but possible side effects, it is recommended that the actual likelihood of severe adverse events be described to help the patient understand the smallness of the risk (though it may be quite difficult for patients to weigh rare side effect risks in proper perspective) [18]. Furthermore, the differences in patients' values regarding efficacy and side effects demonstrate that patient preference is not homogenous. Considering these factors, educating the patient regarding side effects in an explicit and realistic manner and then allowing the patient to make a fully informed decision may be a good approach [11].

14.5.2 Steroid Phobia

The myth of a side effect plays a role in the degree of adherence, and a discussion of patient preferences regarding potential adverse events is prudent. One such modality of treatment that has gained an undeserved reputation is the topical corticosteroid. The collections of falsehoods have supplemented the already worrisome truths regarding steroids such as the potential for changes in skin thickness. The resulting fear is so common, a moniker has arisen: "steroid phobia" [45]. Patient education regarding the methods clinicians use to avoid adverse outcomes from steroids is important, and patients also often feel encouraged when a physician states that monitoring for side effects will occur [3, 8].

14.5.3 The Effect of Age and the Burden of Disease

Variance in a patient's preference regarding trade-offs is influenced by several factors, including the sociodemographics of the patient and the degree of the patient's disease. Younger patients and women tend to place more emphasis on likelihood of benefit, whereas older patients are more concerned about side effects [11]. Teenagers are especially concerned about visible side effects, yet are relatively nonconcerned about side effects such as hepatotoxicity [30]. Additionally, the degree of skin disease influences the patient's preference regarding side effects—for skin diseases that have a significant impact on a patient's life, he or she will be willing to accept even significant adverse events, such as liver damage [7]. Finally, patients with significant comorbidities including heart disease, diabetes mellitus, and depression tend to be more concerned about the side effects of their dermatologic medications [46].

14.6 Conclusion

By engaging patients and allowing them to become partners in the treatment planning process, the dermatologist can optimize aspects of the four principles linked closely with treatment satisfaction and adherence to a treatment regimen: selecting a convenient regimen, choosing the ideal drug vehicle for the patient's lifestyle, balancing efficacy, and minimizing unwanted effects. While understanding the literature aids in awareness of the scenarios in which patients are nonadherent to their treatments, the primary goal is to develop an open, honest relationship with patients so that they feel comfortable directly explaining the difficulties with their current treatment plan.

References

1. Schaarschmidt M-L, Schmieder A, Umar N et al (2011) Patient preferences for psoriasis treatments: process characteristics can outweigh outcome attributes. Arch Dermatol 147(11): 1285–1294
2. Umar N, Schaarschmidt M, Schmieder A, Peitsch W, Schöllgen I, Terris D (2013) Matching physicians' treatment recommendations to patients' treatment preferences is associated with improvement in treatment satisfaction. J Eur Acad Dermatol Venereol 27(6):763–770
3. Brown KK, Rehmus WE, Kimball AB (2006) Determining the relative importance of patient motivations for nonadherence to topical corticosteroid therapy in psoriasis. J Am Acad Dermatol 55(4):607–613
4. Webster GF, Leyden JJ, Gross JA (2013) Comparative pharmacokinetic profiles of a novel isotretinoin formulation (isotretinoin-Lidose) and the innovator isotretinoin formulation: a randomized, 4-treatment, crossover study. J Am Acad Dermatol 69(5):762–767
5. Weinstein GD, White GM (1993) An approach to the treatment of moderate to severe psoriasis with rotational therapy. J Am Acad Dermatol 28(3):454–459
6. Lebwohl M, Menter A, Koo J, Feldman SR (2004) Combination therapy to treat moderate to severe psoriasis. J Am Acad Dermatol 50(3):416–430
7. Ashcroft D, Seston E, Griffiths C (2006) Trade – offs between the benefits and risks of drug treatment for psoriasis: a discrete choice experiment with UK dermatologists. Br J Dermatol 155(6):1236–1241
8. Augustin M, Holland B, Dartsch D, Langenbruch A, Radtke M (2011) Adherence in the treatment of psoriasis: a systematic review. Dermatology 222(4):363–374
9. Webster GF, Leyden JJ, Gross JA (2014) Results of a phase III, double-blind, randomized, parallel-group, non-inferiority study evaluating the safety and efficacy of isotretinoin-Lidose in patients with severe recalcitrant nodular acne. J Drugs Dermatol JDD 13(6):665–670
10. Draelos ZK (1995) Patient compliance: enhancing clinician abilities and strategies. J Am Acad Dermatol 32(5):S42–S48
11. Umar N, Schöllgen I, Terris DD (2011) It is not always about gains: utilities and disutilities associated with treatment features in patients with moderate-to-severe psoriasis. Patient Prefer adherence 6:187–194
12. Lapolla W, Yentzer BA, Bagel J, Halvorson CR, Feldman SR (2011) A review of phototherapy protocols for psoriasis treatment. J Am Acad Dermatol 64(5):936–949
13. Cameron H, Dawe R, Yule S, Murphy J, Ibbotson S, Ferguson J (2002) A randomized, observer – blinded trial of twice vs. three times weekly narrowband ultraviolet B phototherapy for chronic plaque psoriasis. Br J Dermatol 147(5):973–978
14. Fitzmaurice S, Bhutani T, Koo J (2013) Goeckerman regimen for management of psoriasis refractory to biologic therapy: the University of California San Francisco experience. J Am Acad Dermatol 69(4):648–649
15. Fouere S, Adjadj L, Pawin H (2005) How patients experience psoriasis: results from a European survey. J Eur Acad Dermatol Venereol 19(s3):2–6

16. Richards H, Fortune D, Griffiths C (2006) Adherence to treatment in patients with psoriasis. J Eur Acad Dermatol Venereol 20(4):370–379
17. Van de Kerkhof P, De Hoop D, De Korte J, Cobelens S, Kuipers M (2000) Patient compliance and disease management in the treatment of psoriasis in the Netherlands. Dermatology 200(4):292–298
18. Davis SA, Feldman SR (2014) An illustrated dictionary of behavioral economics for healthcare professionals, CreateSpace, Charleston
19. Eisen SA, Miller DK, Woodward RS, Spitznagel E, Przybeck TR (1990) The effect of prescribed daily dose frequency on patient medication compliance. Arch Intern Med 150(9):1881–1884
20. Jones-Caballero M, Unaeze J, Penas PF, Stern RS (2007) Use of biological agents in patients with moderate to severe psoriasis: a cohort-based perspective. Arch Dermatol 143(7): 846–850
21. West C, Narahari S, O'Neill J et al (2013) Adherence to adalimumab in patients with moderate to severe psoriasis. Dermatol Online J 19(5):18182
22. Yentzer BA, Ade RA, Fountain JM et al (2010) Simplifying regimens promotes greater adherence and outcomes with topical acne medications: a randomized controlled trial. Cutis Cutan Med Pract 86(2):103–108
23. Bangalore S, Kamalakkannan G, Parkar S, Messerli FH (2007) Fixed-dose combinations improve medication compliance: a meta-analysis. Am J Med 120(8):713–719
24. Kircik L (2009) Rapid and efficacious fixed-combination monotherapy: desired results for the patient and improved adherence for the clinician. Cutis Cutan Med Pract 84(5 Suppl):5–11
25. Kellett N, West F, Finlay A (2006) Conjoint analysis: a novel, rigorous tool for determining patient preferences for topical antibiotic treatment for acne. A randomised controlled trial. Br J Dermatol 154(3):524–532
26. Longshore SJ, Hollandsworth K (2003) Acne vulgaris: one treatment does not fit all. Cleve Clin J Med 70(8):670–670
27. Del Rosso JQ (2009) A 6% benzoyl peroxide foaming cloth cleanser used in the treatment of acne vulgaris: aesthetic characteristics, patient preference considerations, and impact on compliance with treatment. J Clin Aesth Dermatol 2(7):26
28. Yentzer BA, Wood AA, Sagransky MJ et al (2011) An Internet-based survey and improvement of acne treatment outcomes. Arch Dermatol 147(10):1223–1224
29. Gottlieb AB, Ford RO, Spellman MC (2003) The efficacy and tolerability of clobetasol propionate foam 0.05% in the treatment of mild to moderate plaque-type psoriasis of nonscalp regions. J Cutan Med Surg 7(3):185–192
30. Baldwin HE (2006) Tricks for improving compliance with acne therapy. Dermatol Ther 19(4):224–236
31. Del Rosso JQ (2005) The role of the vehicle in combination acne therapy. Cutis 76(2 Suppl):15–18
32. Dréno B, Thiboutot D, Gollnick H et al (2010) Large – scale worldwide observational study of adherence with acne therapy. Int J Dermatol 49(4):448–456
33. Thiboutot D, Gollnick H, Bettoli V et al (2009) New insights into the management of acne: an update from the Global Alliance to improve outcomes in Acne group. J Am Acad Dermatol 60(5):S1–S50
34. Housman TS, Mellen BG, Rapp SR, Fieischer A, Feldman SR (2002) Patients with psoriasis prefer solution and foam vehicles: a quantitative assessment of vehicle preference. Cutis N Y 70(6):327–334
35. Feldman SR, Housman TS (2003) Patients' vehicle preference for corticosteroid treatments of scalp psoriasis. Am J Clin Dermatol 4(4):221–224
36. Herz G, Blum G, Yawalkar S (1991) Halobetasol propionate cream by day and halobetasol propionate ointment at night for the treatment of pediatric patients with chronic, localized plaque psoriasis and atopic dermatitis. J Am Acad Dermatol 25(6):1166–1169

37. GoodRx [Internet] (2014) Santa Monica: GoodRx, Inc. (Cited 4 Oct 2014). Available from: http://www.goodrx.com/clobetasol
38. UpToDate [internet] (2014) Alphen aan den Rijn, Netherlands: Wolters Kluwer N.V. (Cited 4 Oct 2014). Available from: http://www.uptodate.com/contents/clobetasol-drug-information?source=search_result&search=clobetasol&selectedTitle=1%7E47#F152823
39. Reisfeld PL (2014) How high is up? Generic prices rise. Cutis 93(1):6
40. Schaarschmidt ML, Umar N, Schmieder A et al (2013) Patient preferences for psoriasis treatments: impact of treatment experience. J Eur Acad Dermatol Venereol 27(2):187–198
41. Cook-Bolden F (2006) Subject preferences for acne treatments containing adapalene gel 0.1%: results of the MORE trial. Cutis 78(1 Suppl):26–33
42. Draelos ZD (2008) Improving compliance in acne treatment: benzoyl peroxide considerations. Cutis 82(5 Suppl):17–20
43. Seston EM, Ashcroft DM, Griffiths CE (2007) Balancing the benefits and risks of drug treatment: a stated-preference, discrete choice experiment with patients with psoriasis. Arch Dermatol 143(9):1175–1179
44. Opmeer B, Heydendael V, Deborgie C et al (2007) Patients with moderate-to-severe plaque psoriasis preferred oral therapies to phototherapies: a preference assessment based on clinical scenarios with trade-off questions. J Clin Epidemiol 60(7):696–703
45. Kojima R, Fujiwara T, Matsuda A et al (2013) Factors associated with steroid phobia in caregivers of children with atopic dermatitis. Pediatr Dermatol 30(1):29–35
46. Schmieder A, Schaarschmidt M-L, Umar N et al (2012) Comorbidities significantly impact patients' preferences for psoriasis treatments. J Am Acad Dermatol 67(3):363–372

Chapter 15
Dealing with Forgetfulness

Alyson Snyder and Arash Taheri

How much of poor adherence is due to patients' forgetfulness? It turns out, a substantial portion of patients start using their prescription correctly, but do not consistently use it [1]. In fact, in some studies a quarter of patients cite forgetfulness as their reason for nonadherence [2]. Adherence to medications tends to decrease over time [3]. Some patients discontinue medications and do not use them at all. This is attributed to a variety of reasons discussed in other chapters. Some patients use their medicine inconsistently or incorrectly mainly because they forget to do so.

In order to target the population of patients who forget to use their medications, we must first examine how habits work. It takes a lot of energy to power the brain. In order to conserve energy, our brains try to run as efficiently as possible. One way that our brains are able to become more efficient is by chunking. Chunking is a process by which a sequence of actions is converted into an automatic routine orchestrated by a center in our brains called the basal ganglia [4]. Meaning, the brain tends to combine tasks that it thinks belong together. Our brains store a vast array of chunks ranging from short and simple series, like unlocking the door before reaching to turn the knob, to more lengthy and complex series like the process that a professional musician goes through when tuning their instrument. Chunks become routines, and routines are the roots of habits. But, a habit is more than just a routine. It includes two additional steps. These three steps create the "habit loop" as described in *The Power of Habit* by Charles Duhigg.

A cue or signal begins the loop by alerting the brain that current situations are perfect to execute the specified habit [4]. Then, the routine kicks in whether it's

A. Snyder, BS
OMS-III, Edward Via College of Osteopathic Medicine, Blacksburg, VA, USA
e-mail: asnyder@vcom.vt.edu

A. Taheri (✉)
Departments of Dermatology, Center for Dermatology Research, Wake Forest School of Medicine, Winston-Salem, NC, USA
e-mail: ataheri@wakehealth.edu

© Springer International Publishing Switzerland 2016
S.A. Davis (ed.), *Adherence in Dermatology*,
DOI 10.1007/978-3-319-30994-1_15

emotional, mental, or physical [4]. Lastly, there is a reward that makes the habit worth creating and continuing in the future [4]. Of course, practice makes perfect. Eventually, habits become second nature. A craving ultimately forms to keep them going [4]. The word *craving* makes one think that there is an overt desire to continue the routine by conveying images of drug addicts, but actually the reward has the most powerful impact and the craving may be a completely subconscious result. For instance, someone will continue to arrive to work every morning despite hating their job (the routine) because they subconsciously crave the reward, in this case the paycheck.

Now, let us walk through an example. People tend to look both ways before crossing the street. The cue would be approaching the end of a sidewalk. The routine would be to look both ways and the reward would be safe passage. These habits become so instilled that when later presented with the same conditions, our brains will automatically revert to the original habit [4]. Deviation from any of these elements (i.e., the exact same cue, routine, and reward) will not evoke the same habit [4]. For example, if every morning you go to exercise at the gym near your place of work and that gym closes 1 day to move to a larger building somewhere else, you are likely to stop going to the gym because the cue in the habit loop is gone.

Now that we have a better understanding of how habits work, let us learn how to form and change our own habits. Duhigg provides an approach to shaping our own habits using the following steps:

1. Identify the routine.
2. Experiment with rewards.
3. Isolate a cue.
4. Have a plan.

In the context of medicine, here is a scenario where a patient needs to create a habit in order to apply a topical cream to the face once in the morning and once at night for acne treatment. The routine is simple, applying the medication. Then, one must experiment with rewards such as noticeable skin improvements, a feeling of being in control of one's condition, or better self-esteem. After completing the routine with each new reward, write down three things that come to mind. Later reviewing what was written about each reward will help determine which reward will provide enough incentive or craving to continue. Next, identify a cue that will prompt the routine, like an alarm, placing the medicine in a particular spot, or leaving reminder notes. To better isolate an appropriate cue, write down the location, time, feeling, if other people were involved, and the immediately preceding action surrounding the completed routine. In this way one will be able to isolate exactly what triggered the routine before or what caused a deviation from the routine before. There must be an understanding of the cue or else one might choose the wrong remedy. If a particular stressor is the reason a patient forgets to apply their medication, then adding a reminder note may be pointless if the patient does not realize that the stressor fuels them to forget the medication. A more in-depth discussion of cues will take place later in this chapter. Putting it all together gives a plan, a note on the medicine cabinet cues the routine of applying the medication, and the renewed self-esteem encourages the process.

The following sections address each major group of reminder strategies and any supporting research. Reminders represent cues discussed above.

15.1 Text Messages

Text messaging has taken communication by storm. The younger population is a particular target of this intervention, as they are some of the heaviest users of text messaging. The majority of reminder-based research has involved experimenting with text messaging. A randomized controlled trial by Armstrong et al. sent half of the participants' daily text messages displaying the weather and a reminder to apply sunscreen [5]. Electronic monitors on sunscreen tubes recorded use. After a 6-week period, there was almost 30 % higher adherence in sunscreen use in those receiving text messages compared to control, and 69 % of the test group said they would continue to use the text message reminders [5]. Another trial sent daily reminder and educational text messages to psoriasis patients for 12 weeks resulted in significantly better adherence and improved disease and quality of life assessed by professional indexes in respect to the control [6]. Meta-analyses reviewing text message reminders in dermatologic and other specialties have shown significant improvement in medication adherence [5, 7, 8]. Text messaging is cheap, customizable, and efficient, and as accessibility and popularity continues, so will the utility of text messaging for reminding patients.

15.2 Phone/Voice Messages

Automated voice messages are one of the oldest forms of reminders used by medical professionals, but have traditionally been used for appointment date or refill reminders instead of medication adherence reminders. Being automated makes them easy to deploy, and calls are more wide reaching than text messages since they can reach landlines as well as cell phones. However, they are less customizable and suffer from more glitches such as incorrect time of calls and voice recognition difficulties [9]. Despite these issues, a literature review by Biem et al. demonstrated that voice reminders are associated with better adherence to medication in areas of preventative medicine and chronic conditions [10].

15.3 Apps

In the revolution of smartphones, tablets, and wireless Internet, the phrase "there's an app for that" is not a joke. A quick search on the App Store will reap results of apps that are designed for the sole purpose of reminding people to take their medication(s). These programs allow for complete customization. For instance, just the type of alert has multiple options such as text, email, sound, image, voice, and others. Other app features also allow for medication tracking, alerting you when your medications are running low and providing you with a printed log of when each medication was used/taken. Software is typically inexpensive. Providers could even make their own. Web-based services are another option for electronic-based reminders. Again, most sites provide links between other methods of communication like email. Providers can also create their own web pages and web apps. A review of four randomized controlled trials by Chanhyun Park et al. found a positive effect on acne medication adherence in groups that participated in periodic web-based health education tools compared to groups using another technology-based intervention [11]. Apps show promise as their innovation, popularity, and accessibility continues to increase.

15.4   Alarms

Alarm clocks are a much older technology that have evolved with the times and assimilated into watches and cell phones. Alarms on cell phones allow each patient to customize reminders from the time that it triggers to the sound. Alarms also include an active component to turn the reminder off.

15.5   Pill Organizers

Pill boxes are nothing new, but they are a great way to keep pills organized. Convenient and simple, you only have to fill them once a week or even once a month depending on the size. Now, pharmacies also offer pill blister packaging. Heneghan et al. evaluated eight studies involving 1,137 participants who were already taking medications for at least 1 month [12]. Regardless of who is doing the assembling, the type of packaging, the medication, and the health problem, reminder packaging demonstrated a significant increase in medication adherence measured by pill counts [12]. The obvious downfall for dermatology is that it cannot accommodate other types of medications such as ointments or creams.

15.6   Tie to Daily Routine

Making medication use part of the individual's daily routine seems elementary, but is very difficult in practice. After all, it was not long ago that most adults decided to start brushing their teeth twice daily. It takes real mental power and repetition to add something to a daily routine and keep it there. One strategy that may help integrate medication adherence into the daily routine is medication placement. The location of the medication may be dictated by the dosage instructions. For example, if the medication is to be taken three times a day, once in the morning, once midday, and once at night, one could simply separate the prescription into separate containers and place one container by the toothbrush, one at work, and one on the bedside table so that each dose easily fit into one's lifestyle, and there is a visual reminder. Creams and medications of other mediums may also be separated in order to provide practicality as long as safety precautions are met.

15.7 Recording When the Medication Is Taken

Keeping a record of every time a medication is used not only provides the physician with a document of the patient's adherence (if being truthful) but may also create a habit of its own. There are numerous means by which one can record use, such as tally marks or marking dates on a calendar. There is little data to speak of the efficacy of this reminder system.

15.8 Notes for Self

Another common and classic method of reminders is to leave visible written notes or signs for oneself. We have an iconic image of someone who has notes strung up all over their work space. Instead of creating a cluttered environment, placing a single note where the medication will be used (like the bathroom) or where the medication is stored (like the refrigerator) will aid in incorporating medication use into the daily routine and forming a habit. Thanks to the advent of sticky notes and multiple different adhesives, notes can be customized in content, look, and location.

15.9 Ask Someone Else to Remind You

Placing the responsibility of remembering onto another person may be a good choice for children or elderly, both of whom cannot remember and have difficulty performing activities of daily living on their own. There is still a problem though when the patient is not willing to listen to the person delivering the reminder or the person doing the reminding forgets. A study comparing adherence strategies to topical acne medication among teenagers found that the parental reminder group had the worst adherence [13].

15.10 Written Action Plan

Many patients may have poor adherence to medication not simply because they forget to use the medication, but because they forget *how* to use the medication. Written action plans (WAPs) were historically used for the parents of pediatric asthmatics to navigate through the appropriate treatment plan [1]. WAPs have a promising role in other diseases especially in dermatology where there are confusing and complicating treatment regimens like atopic dermatitis and psoriasis [1]. A study by Rork et al. gathering the parents' opinions of eczema action plans found that an overwhelming majority of parents (86%) found the action plans helpful in treatment [14]. While Rork's study cannot conclude that the eczema action plans directly lead to eczema recovery, more than half (68%) of the parents whose child's eczema improved partially attributed the success to the action plan [14].

No one of the mentioned intervention strategies has been shown to be totally effective (Fig. 15.1). The majority of interventions are moderately successful. Combining these strategies with each other and adding them to other interventions can help with achieving the best adherence to medications.

Forgetfulness is the chief reason a considerable proportion of patients cite non-adherence to medication. Charles Duhigg's book *The Power of Habit* explores how and why we are able to form, change, and break habits. The "habit loop" made up of a cue, routine, and reward is the piece of a habit. The cue can be targeted by reminder strategies to hopefully help the forgetful patients become more adherent to their medications. There are many reminder strategies to choose from on a personal or provider level to increase adherence due to forgetfulness. A lot of the newer modalities like text messaging hint at success and bursting popularity. Older strategies, including pill boxes, have stood up to the test again resulting in increased medication adherence. Unfortunately, there is no single technique or algorithm to

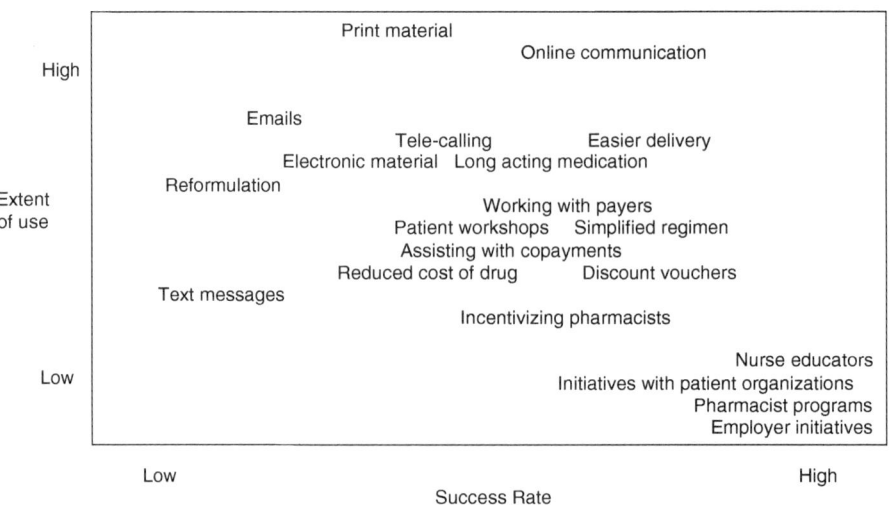

Fig. 15.1 Extent of use vs. success rate of sample interventions as ranked by respondents [15]. This is the result of interviews with 66 life science executives representing pharmaceutical and biotech manufacturers, payers, pharmacists, patients, and advocacy groups, across Denmark, France, Germany, the Netherlands, Portugal, Spain, Switzerland, the United Kingdom, and the United States

employ to determine which reminder strategy would work best for a particular patient. Patients usually engage in a process of trial and error, try multiple ways, or combine multiple strategies to find a method that ultimately works for them.

References

1. Feldman SR (2008) Practical ways to improve patients' treatment outcomes, 1st edn. Medical Quality Enhancement Corp, Winston Salem
2. Nonadherence: tools for combating persistence and compliance issues. Frost & Sullivan 2005. Available from: URL: http://www.buppractice.com/node/5354
3. Blaschke TF, Osterberg L, Vrijens B, Urquhart J (2012) Adherence to medications: insights arising from studies on the unreliable link between prescribed and actual drug dosing histories. Annu Rev Pharmacol Toxicol 52:275–301
4. Duhigg C (2012) The power of habit: why we do what we do in life and business. Random House, New York
5. Armstrong AW, Watson AJ, Makredes M, Frangos JE, Kimball AB, Kvedar JC (2009) Text-message reminders to improve sunscreen use: a randomized, controlled trial using electronic monitoring. Arch Dermatol 145(11):1230–1236
6. Balato N, Megna M, Di CL, Balato A, Ayala F (2013) Educational and motivational support service: a pilot study for mobile-phone-based interventions in patients with psoriasis. Br J Dermatol 168(1):201–205
7. Fenerty SD, West C, Davis SA, Kaplan SG, Feldman SR (2012) The effect of reminder systems on patients' adherence to treatment. Patient Prefer Adherence 6:127–135
8. Vervloet M, Linn AJ, van Weert JC, de Bakker DH, Bouvy ML, van DL (2012) The effectiveness of interventions using electronic reminders to improve adherence to chronic medication: a systematic review of the literature. J Am Med Inform Assoc 19(5):696–704
9. Reidel K, Tamblyn R, Patel V, Huang A (2008) Pilot study of an interactive voice response system to improve medication refill compliance. BMC Med Inform Decis Mak 8:46
10. Biem HJ, Turnell RW, D'Arcy C (2003) Computer telephony: automated calls for medical care. Clin Invest Med 26(5):259–268
11. Park C, Kim G, Patel I, Chang J, Tan X (2014) Improving adherence to acne treatment: the emerging role of application software. Clin Cosmet Investig Dermatol 7:65–72
12. Heneghan CJ, Glasziou P, Perera R (2006) Reminder packaging for improving adherence to self-administered long-term medications. Cochrane Database Syst Rev (1):CD005025
13. Yentzer BA, Gosnell AL, Clark AR, Pearce DJ, Balkrishnan R, Camacho FT et al (2011) A randomized controlled pilot study of strategies to increase adherence in teenagers with acne vulgaris. J Am Acad Dermatol 64(4):793–795
14. Rork JF, Sheehan WJ, Gaffin JM, Timmons KG, Sidbury R, Schneider LC et al (2012) Parental response to written eczema action plans in children with eczema. Arch Dermatol 148(3):391–392
15. Patient adherence: the next frontier in patient care. Capgemini Consulting 2011 [cited 5 May 2014]; Available from: URL: http://www.capgemini.com/resource-file-access/resource/pdf/Patient_Adherence__The_Next_Frontier_in_Patient_Care.pdf

Chapter 16
Building Motivation and Self-Efficacy

Scott A. Davis

Some patients still struggle with taking their medications even after a good physician-patient relationship has been established, an appropriate medication has been chosen, and steps have been taken to minimize forgetfulness. These patients may still not be motivated to take the medication, or may lack the belief in their own ability to achieve the desired adherence behaviors or clinical outcomes. The information-motivation-behavioral skills model [1] suggests that both motivation and self-efficacy have a crucial influence on behavioral skills, which then produce better adherence behavior. This chapter will explore motivational interviewing for building motivation, some techniques for improving self-efficacy, and an example of a practical technology-based intervention that illustrates many of the principles presented.

16.1 Motivational Interviewing

Motivational interviewing (MI) is a widely used, patient-centered approach for facilitating behavior change, including improvement of adherence to treatment [2, 3]. Like many forms of psychotherapy, MI involves meeting the patient at whatever point they may be on their journey. Some patients might actually be in a precontemplative stage of behavior change, where they have not truly started to think about changing their behavior [4]. Others may have reached a contemplative stage, where they are ready to think about changing the behavior, but not firmly committed to a

S.A. Davis
Department of Dermatology, Wake Forest School of Medicine, Winston-Salem, NC, USA

Division of Pharmaceutical Outcomes and Policy, University of North Carolina Eshelman
School of Pharmacy, Chapel Hill, NC, USA
e-mail: sdavis81@email.unc.edu

© Springer International Publishing Switzerland 2016   171
S.A. Davis (ed.), *Adherence in Dermatology*,
DOI 10.1007/978-3-319-30994-1_16

plan to do so. Others may have already made a serious effort to change the behavior, but then relapsed into the old behavior pattern. By understanding where they are in their thinking process, and what tends to motivate them more generally, we can help patients achieve positive changes in their adherence behavior.

In behavioral economics, the generation effect refers to the tendency to be more likely to remember or believe ideas that are perceived as self-generated, rather than suggested by someone else [5]. Similar to psychotherapy, a clinician using MI will want to take advantage of the generation effect to induce the patient to talk him/herself into the healthy behavior. Areas of ambivalence can be highlighted and used to set goals. For example, patients with severe lupus erythematosus can be asked what activities they are not able to do on account of their lupus. If a patient says she would really like to be able to spend time outdoors with her energetic young children, then we can tell that an approach that enables this activity would probably be well received by this patient. By gently exposing the conflict between the patient's expressed preference to enjoy freedom from disability and her behavior of not taking her lupus medication, we may be able to generate newfound motivation to resolve the discrepancy by being more adherent to the medication.

Guiding is the ideal to strive for when performing MI, avoiding the ineffective extremes of passive following or authoritarian directing [2, 6]. Passive following might tend not to evoke reasons favoring behavior change and might therefore result in a missed opportunity to demonstrate why the patient should want to change. In a series of videos, MI coinventor Stephen Rollnick models the two failed approaches vs. the successful approach in smoking cessation [7]. The passive approach strikes me as showing exactly what a clinician should do if he or she wanted to use MI to get the patient to keep smoking. It seems very empathetic, but causes the patient to verbalize all the reasons that he would not want to give up smoking. At the end, the patient appears firmly convinced that smoking is an essential stress reducer in his life, and thus the reasons to keep smoking outweigh the reasons to quit.

On the other hand, authoritarian directing tends to assume that the patient is willing to follow in any direction the clinician might want, which is generally not the case [6]. Even if the patient is too timid to openly oppose the clinician's plan, he or she is likely to come back the next time with the same adherence problem or maybe even find a different physician who is more empathetic. Patients may not feel competent to win an argument with their physician, but in the privacy of their own home, they will exercise their veto power over the unacceptable treatment plan by not adhering. Just as many of us will say, "You can't make me do it!" when our spouse asks us to take out the trash, patients will resist ideas that appear to reflect a dominant clinician ignoring their values. For more discussion of this phenomenon, see Chaps. 11 and 12 in *An Illustrated Dictionary of Behavioral Economics for Healthcare Professionals* [8].

An important skill in successfully conducting MI is the elicit-provide-elicit technique. In the video modeling successful technique, Rollnick creates an opening to provide information on smoking cessation by asking what the patient knows about ways to quit smoking [7]. Without appropriate preparation, it would have been difficult to tell whether the patient was ready to receive this information, and the patient might have been offended by the unsolicited information, similar to most people's reaction upon receiving spam messages. In the case of medication adherence, begin by asking what the patient knows about medications for their condition. It is recommended to respond with a reflective statement, such as "It sounds like you are concerned about side effects of fluocinonide for psoriasis. You have heard that it is a steroid, and you are concerned about the side effects of this class of medications." Next, ask permission to give the information: "Would it be OK if I shared some information about side effects of psoriasis treatments?" If the patient says yes, continue with something like, "You're right, the medications you described have quite a few side effects, such as (whatever the patient said). Many of my patients who are concerned about side effects have tried a natural vitamin D product, which has fewer side effects. Does that sound like something you think you might be interested in?"

16.2 Improving Self-Efficacy

Self-efficacy is patients' belief in their ability to accomplish a task, such as taking their medication as directed. Besides motivation, self-efficacy is the other main determinant of behavioral skills, and hence adherence, in the IMB model [1]. Barriers to patients' confidence in their ability to take medication may include cost, medication access, time or disruption to routine, or lack of knowledge about how to take the medication. Some patients are very frank about experiencing these barriers, but many are not. A way to open discussion of barriers to self-efficacy is to say something like, "On a scale of 1 to 10, where 1 is least confident and 10 is most confident, how confident are you in your ability to take your medications?" [9] If the answer is a 6, first ask, "Why not a 4?" to allow the patient to express some reasons for optimism. Then ask, "Why not an 8?" or "What would it take to get you to a 9 or a 10?" to gather information on possible barriers [9].

Cost is a very common barrier, and many patients are reluctant to admit that they have difficulties with affording their medications. Given the very high cost of many medications and wide variability in insurance coverage, inquiring about cost-related barriers is critical. Many pharmaceutical companies offer discount cards, and patients may be surprised to find that they often do not even have to prove they are needy to qualify. Free samples can also be a way to allow patients to try a product for a short time without incurring substantial cost. Most states also have programs to assist low-income patients with finding affordable sources of medications, so it is helpful to have the contact information for these programs readily available. In one pilot study, patients had the ability to watch a series of educational videos on aspects of diabetes self-management, and there was a decline from 65 % at baseline to 34 % at follow-up in the number agreeing with the statement "It's hard for me to pay for my glucose monitoring supplies" [10]. This finding suggests that many patients are not aware of the availability of programs that can help with cost-related barriers, but only need a little additional information to overcome financial issues with adherence.

Access to treatment is another important barrier and can include logistical issues with transportation to the clinic or the pharmacy. Transportation is an especially important issue when prescribing repeated sessions of treatments such as office phototherapy [11]. A home light unit [12], judicious use of tanning beds, or spending more time in the sun may help patients who live far from the nearest phototherapy center [13]. As with cost, most states have programs to assist with transportation for medical needs, including transportation to the pharmacy. Patients can also be encouraged to sign up for mail-order prescriptions when possible.

Time is another major barrier to self-efficacy, especially with topical dermatological treatments that must be applied multiple times daily for large areas of the body. Asking about how treatment use disrupts the patient's routine is a good way to determine whether lack of time is affecting adherence. Offering a very short course of treatment, such as a 3-day regimen of twice-a-day scalp psoriasis treatment, may increase patients' willingness to adhere to the regimen [14]. Patients can come in for a return visit at 3 days or be directed to call the physician's cell phone to report how they are doing. If they can use the medication well for 3 days, they may be amazed at their improvement and be empowered to believe they can incorporate medication use into their busy day in the future [14].

Patients also suffer low self-efficacy if they do not know how to use the medication properly. Injectable biologics are perhaps the most obvious dermatologic example, but topical medications are also subject to widespread underdosing [15], making patients feel puzzled when they do not see the expected improvement. Demonstrating exactly how the medication should be taken, and providing written materials to enhance retention of knowledge, is usually helpful – even if we think the patient already knows. Asking patients to demonstrate their technique for taking their medication can help identify errors, or else elicit an honest confession of "I don't know what I'm supposed to do." Written action plans for complex regimens can reduce the patient's need to remember everything they have been told during the office visit [14, 16].

16.3   Example: Causa Research and an Internet Survey Approach

Causa Research was formed in 2012 to develop a patented system for using frequent online contact to improve adherence by mimicking the effect of extra office visits. As discussed in previous chapters, using weekly Internet surveys with a small incentive for participation (the incentive was not specifically tied to adherence) increased mean adherence to 89 % in the intervention group, compared to 33 % in the control group [17]. This approach was more successful than some reminder approaches, which may fail because they assume a certain degree of motivation is already present [18]. Reflecting the emotions generated by unwanted and overly intrusive reminder devices, reports abound of patients crushing their loud, annoying reminder devices under the wheels of their cars [19]. The Internet survey approach is designed to meet the need for a subtler method that would be perceived positively by most patients.

The primary aim of this approach is to produce a deliberate Hawthorne effect on adherence [20]. The Hawthorne effect comes from a study in which factory workers who were being observed showed greater productivity. It proved impossible to conduct a study that merely observed workers' productivity without modifying their behavior [21]. Similarly, clinical trials have frequent visits so that patients' clinical outcomes can be assessed at many time points, such as 1, 2, 4, 6, 8, and 12 weeks instead of only 6 and 12 weeks in usual care. Although the purpose of the visits is not specifically to improve adherence, clinical trials do tend to display better adherence to treatment. Patients do not want to disappoint their physicians, so they start taking their medication a few days before the visit ("white-coat" adherence) [22], similar to how people start flossing a few days before going to the dentist. If the visits are frequent enough, patients may never experience a long period of nonadherence. Building on these observations, further studies were performed to demonstrate that intentionally adding a single extra office visit at 1 week successfully improves adherence [23]. Adding visits on a typical clinical trial schedule for acne patients improved adherence, while reminding patients or their parents with daily phone calls produced neutral or negative effects [24].

The Internet survey approach also builds on the behavioral economics concept of a nudge. According to Thaler and Sunstein in their book *Nudge*, a nudge is a design feature that can be built into a system to shift user preferences slightly in an unobtrusive fashion [25]. The user tends to do what is obvious within the design of the system, such as buying more grocery items that are placed at eye level or at the checkout while avoiding items that are on the bottom shelf. By using nudges, the designer is able to modify the user's choices without the user even realizing that the design feature is being employed. However, a nudge must not become a "shove" [25], or it tends to evoke a hostile response called reactance [26]. For example, a Mongolian barbeque might try to nudge customers into only getting a limited amount of food since it is more profitable when customers do not take full advantage of the all-you-can-eat aspect. However, a hungry customer might come in and notice that the service seems intentionally slow, so that it takes far too long to go back to the grill as many times as the customer wanted. The customer would begin to suspect that the restaurant is employing a manipulative tactic to avoid providing the amount of value expected and would feel resentful. The customer would feel shoved into eating less, rather than nudged. Similarly, medication reminders would tend to be perceived as a shove unless the patient is already fairly motivated and only needs help with remembering to take the medication.

To mimic the effects of an extra office visit without the time burden of an in-person consultation, the Internet survey approach asks patients to answer a few questions that are similar to what they would be asked at a regular visit. These include how difficult it is to take the medication, how effective they think the medication is, how many times the medication was used, how severe their disease is now, and what side effects they have experienced. A picture of their smiling physician communicates caring and portrays the online survey as an extension of the friendly guidance that patients receive at their usual visit. Customization of the survey can involve adding questions designed to elicit specific thought processes. For example, asking "What time do you take the medication each day?" suggests to patients that they should strive for a routine where they take the medication at the same time each day. Phrasing the suggestion as an open-ended question is less threatening and consistent with the spirit of gently nudging patients in the right direction. Even if it does not matter what time the medication is taken, establishing a routine is likely to lead to more consistent use.

After a few weeks, the survey is intended to generate regular habits of medication use. Telling the patient that they will receive a survey at 1 week creates a default option of filling the prescription immediately, rather than procrastinating. Thus, the survey approach is designed to minimize primary nonadherence and causes patients to start the treatment regimen on time. A trial currently in progress is designed to determine whether the survey can be given less often after an initial period of establishing adherent habits. This trial consists of four arms – three intervention arms and a control arm. In all three intervention arms, patients receive the survey weekly for the first 8 weeks, but then one arm continues receiving the survey weekly up to 12 months, one arm receives it monthly, and one arm stops receiving surveys.

16.4   Conclusion

Motivational interviewing, addressing barriers to self-efficacy, and frequent contact to mimic office visits are just a few techniques to achieve the goal of maximizing adherence in patients who are not sure they have the desire or ability to follow the regimen optimally. To summarize the results of the last few chapters on methods to improve adherence:

• Optimize the physician-patient relationship by sending the right message and showing how much you care. Many other strategies for improving adherence presuppose a strong, trusting relationship with the patient. These strategies then use that relationship as a foundation to persuade the patient to follow through with the regimen.
• Choose a treatment that the patient is willing to use. Ideally, the treatment should be convenient with no more than once-a-day dosing, and feature a vehicle that is not messy or irritating. Unnecessary complexity, especially prescribing multiple products when the patient has not previously been adherent, should be avoided whenever possible. When possible, explain predictable side effects as a sign that the treatment is working.
• Assess forgetfulness by asking about the patient's routine, and offer solutions that make it easier to remember to take the medication every day. Strive to automate habits, so they become embedded within the brain's automatic system of behavior. Use aids such as pill boxes or reminder apps to facilitate regular daily medication use.

- Build motivation and self-efficacy using principles of motivational interviewing and uncovering deficits in affordability, access, time, and knowledge that may interfere with medication adherence. Use white-coat adherence to your advantage, and direct the patient toward positive behavior using gentle nudges, not shoves.

The art of modifying patients' adherence behavior still has a long way to go, but this book should provide some practical tools that all clinicians can use to get started. With the increased importance of demonstrating quality of care, the importance of using effective adherence-enhancing strategies will only continue to grow over time. We should all continue educating ourselves on the latest new technologies, formulations, and behavioral strategies as they are invented, as the field of adherence contains much still to discover in the future.

References

1. Fisher JD, Fisher WA, Amico KR, Harman JJ (2006) An information-motivation-behavioral skills model of adherence to antiretroviral therapy. Health Psychol 25(4):462–473
2. Miller WR, Rollnick S (2002) Motivational interviewing: preparing people for change, 2nd edn. Guilford, New York
3. Spoelstra SL, Schueller M, Hilton M, Ridenour K (2014) Interventions combining motivational interviewing and cognitive behaviour to promote medication adherence: a literature review. J Clin Nurs 24:1163–1173
4. Prochaska JO, DiClemente CC (1992) Stages of change in the modification of problem behaviors. Prog Behav Modif 28:183–218
5. Dewinstanley PA, Bjork EL (2004) Processing strategies and the generation effect. Mem Cogn 32(6):945–955
6. Rollnick S, Butler CC, Kinnersley P et al (2010) Motivational interviewing. BMJ 340:c1900
7. Miller WR, Moyers TB, Rollnick S (2013) Motivational interviewing: helping people change [DVD or streaming]. Change Companies, Carson, USA, Retrieved from https://www.change-companies.net/motivational_interviewing.php. Accessed 29 Dec 2015
8. Davis SA, Feldman SR (2014) An illustrated dictionary of behavioral economics for healthcare professionals. CreateSpace, Charleston
9. Ogedegbe G, Schoenthaler A, Richardson T et al (2007) An RCT of the effect of motivational interviewing on medication adherence in hypertensive African Americans: rationale and design. Contemp Clin Trials 28:169–181
10. Davis SA, Carpenter DM, Cummings DM et al (2015) Patient adoption of an Internet based diabetes medication tool to improve adherence: a pilot study. International Conference on Communication in Healthcare. New Orleans. 26 Oct
11. Yentzer BA, Gustafson CJ, Feldman SR (2013) Explicit and implicit copayments for phototherapy: examining the cost of commuting. Dermatol Online J 19(6):18563
12. Anderson KL, Feldman SR (2015) A guide to prescribing home phototherapy for patients with psoriasis: the appropriate patient, the type of unit, the treatment regimen, and the potential obstacles. J Am Acad Dermatol 72(5):868–878
13. Radack KP, Farhangian ME, Anderson KL, Feldman SR (2015) A review of the use of tanning beds as a dermatological treatment. Dermatol Ther (Heidelb) 5(1):37–51
14. Feldman SR (2009) Practical ways to improve patients' treatment outcomes. Medical Quality Enhancement Corporation, Winston-Salem

15. Storm A, Benfeldt E, Andersen SE, Serup J (2008) A prospective study of patient adherence to topical treatments: 95% of patients underdose. J Am Acad Dermatol 59(6):975–980
16. Ntuen E, Taylor SL, Kinney M et al (2010) Physicians' perceptions of an eczema action plan for atopic dermatitis. J Dermatol Treat 21(1):28–33
17. Yentzer BA, Gosnell AL, Clark AR et al (2011) A randomized controlled pilot study of strategies to increase adherence in teenagers with acne vulgaris. J Am Acad Dermatol 64(4):793–795
18. Fenerty SD, West C, Davis SA, Kaplan SG, Feldman SR (2012) The effect of reminder systems on patients' adherence to treatment. Patient Prefer Adherence 6:127–135
19. Vander Stichele R (2013) Jean-Michel Metry lecture. European society for patient adherence, compliance, and persistence. Budapest. 15 Nov
20. Davis SA, Feldman SR (2013) Using Hawthorne effects to improve adherence in clinical practice: lessons from clinical trials. JAMA Dermatol 149(4):490–491
21. Glenn C, McMichael A, Feldman SR (2012) Measuring patient satisfaction changes patient satisfaction. J Dermatol Treat 23(2):81–82
22. Feinstein AR (1990) On white-coat effects and the electronic monitoring of compliance. Arch Intern Med 150(7):1377–1378
23. Sagransky MJ, Yentzer BA, Williams LL et al (2010) A randomized controlled pilot study of the effects of an extra office visit on adherence and outcomes in atopic dermatitis. Arch Dermatol 146(12):1428–1430
24. Yentzer BA, Wood AA, Sagransky MJ et al (2011) An internet-based survey and improvement of acne treatment outcomes. Arch Dermatol 147(10):1223–1224
25. Thaler RH, Sunstein CR (2009) Nudge: improving decisions about health, wealth, and happiness, revised and expanded edition. Penguin, New York
26. Dillard JP, Shen L (2005) On the nature of reactance and its role in persuasive health communication. Commun Monogr 72(2):144–168